Schools as a Lens for Understanding the Opioid Epidemic

This book investigates the profound and complex impact of the opioid epidemic on schools in the United States, focusing on diverse aspects such as its history, legislative responses, trends, and implications for students, educators, and schools.

Sharing research from multiple case studies in elementary schools located in Northeast opioid-crisis regions, the book explores the ripple effects of students' adverse childhood experiences, community and household opioid exposure, transiency, homelessness, attendance, as well as the profound struggles of educators dealing with secondary trauma. Shedding light on the untold stories of young children contending with the consequences of opioid exposure, it foregrounds these voices and stories through the unique perspectives of educators. Additionally, the book examines the developing landscape of initiatives to mitigate the crises' effects on students, emphasizing the need for comprehensive approaches. Finally, the book explores potential interventions and strategies to address the complex issues arising from the opioid epidemic in schools, advocating for a comprehensive, multi-tiered approach involving collaboration among various stakeholders.

Through a synthesis of historical context, multiple case studies, qualitative follow-up investigations, and analysis, this book provides a comprehensive understanding of the interconnected challenges posed by the overwhelming impact of the opioid epidemic on education in the United States. It will appeal to scholars, researchers, educational leaders, school administrators, teachers, and post-graduate students with interests in crises education, educational psychology, trauma studies, public health policy, sociology of education, and addiction and substance abuse.

Kathryn A. Welby is Assistant Professor of Education in the Winston School of Education and Social Policy at Merrimack College, the United States.

Routledge Research in Crises Education

This is a series that offers a global platform to engage scholars in continuous academic debate on key challenges and the latest thinking on issues in the fast-growing field of Crises Education. Books in this series could address, but are not limited to, education in the context of natural disasters, warfare, public health crises, refugee and migrant crises, and political and economic crises.

Titles in the series include:

Schools as a Lens for Understanding the Opioid Epidemic
Impacts on Students and Educators in Crisis
Kathryn A. Welby

Schools as a Lens for Understanding the Opioid Epidemic

Impacts on Students and Educators in Crisis

Kathryn A. Welby

Routledge
Taylor & Francis Group
NEW YORK AND LONDON

First published 2025
by Routledge
605 Third Avenue, New York, NY 10158

and by Routledge
4 Park Square, Milton Park, Abingdon, Oxon, OX14 4RN

Routledge is an imprint of the Taylor & Francis Group, an informa business

ISBN: 978-1-032-45675-1 (hbk)
ISBN: 978-1-032-45676-8 (pbk)
ISBN: 978-1-003-37820-4 (ebk)

DOI: 10.4324/9781003378204

Typeset in ITC Galliard Pro
by Apex CoVantage, LLC

To the courageous children and resilient educators touched by the opioid epidemic – your bravery ignites hope

Contents

Prelude

Thoughts from the Field Journal:

At 11:42, I was in Mary's office, eagerly awaiting our scheduled interview. While waiting, I glanced out the window to observe the bustling activity outside. Among the crowd, two men engaged in a conversation while both leaning against a building directly across the street. Although I could not make out their words, a disagreement seemed to suddenly erupt between them. Within moments, it escalated into a physical altercation – punches thrown, bloodshed, a torn sweatshirt, and a shattered glass bottle. Onlookers swiftly dispersed from the scene as chaos ensued. The afternoon's calm was shattered even more so by blaring sirens and the arrival of police cars, their red and blue lights painting the street and shining inside Mary's window. Remarkably, within minutes, the police and the men parted ways without any arrests. It all unraveled within the 20 minutes while I waited for Mary.

The incident lingered in my thoughts, leaving a trail of questions. What sparked the fight? Did Mary see this while outside at recess duty? Even worse, did the students witness it? Are we safe here? Why does no one else in the office area seem disturbed? Mary's secretary is here too, and she did not even look up, continuing her work unfazed. I started to wonder if this is a frequent occurrence.

Mary returned from lunch and recess duty, and the semi-structured interview began. During the interview, I asked a direct yet open-ended question, "How does the opioid epidemic affect your school?"

Her response:

> Look outside this window! This is a direct impact. We all see adults using and dealing all day long. See that window? Somebody leaves drugs on that window, and then somebody else comes and picks it up. I see people right there (pointing outside her window) shooting up heroin. Unfortunately, our young children here are watching this, too.

Mary's words ignited a whirlwind of thoughts, and my mind returned to the altercation. Was the altercation linked to drugs? Money? Respect? The vivid memory of the incident refused to fade.

Later that day, I connected with Jon, a clinical social worker who worked with Mary. Despite our initial in-person meeting being canceled due to a school emergency, we settled for a phone interview.

During our 90-minute conversation, I asked the same question, "How does the opioid epidemic affect your school?"

He responds:

> Students are being schooled in areas in which students, parents, teachers, and staff have to walk over used needles in the streets and sidewalks to get to school. Students are watching people shoot up in their cars outside the classrooms and pass out. People urinate outside classroom windows. . . . Middle schoolers used to put signs in the window saying, "This is a school. Don't smoke or whatever here." "This is a school, don't urinate here." Within the square block of the school . . . we were losing one person a day to a heroin overdose.

The following day, I returned to the same school to meet with Matt, another social worker.

Matt's office windows are covered with student work, such as drawings, paintings, and quotes about grit and resilience. Students could not see outside while in his office, and neither could I. As I sat there looking around his office, I began to think about Mary and Jon's interview, my observation of an altercation, and understand the possible reason the strategically decorated windows block out the daylight.

I asked Matt the same question, "How does the opioid epidemic impact your school?"

Matt's response was, "You can just see it outside. Unfortunately, students look out the window and can see the people that are floridly psychotic, drug-addicted, and the people that are preying on those people."

As I drove home from an eventful week in Maine, recollections of Mary, Jon, and Matt's responses brought me back to my lingering thoughts of the fight observed from the school window. It made me think about the events the students observe daily from their desks, and I wondered about the lasting impacts on the students who witness such distressing events regularly.

Children and educators face profound challenges daily in communities overwhelmed by opioid addiction. Shocking developments continue to unfold regarding the impact on schools, educators, and children in regions significantly affected by the opioid crisis. The present situations and experiences uncovered in this research will affect the future of children, educators, and schools in ways we have yet to completely understand.

January 2019
Maine

Acknowledgment

My heartfelt gratitude goes out to the incredible support system and the individuals who played a pivotal role in bringing this research and book to completion.

I want to acknowledge Merrimack College and its Strategic Academic Research Trajectory (START) program for the time, funds, and mentorship to complete this research and the resultant book – a special mention to Dr. April Bowling, whose leadership and guidance were invaluable throughout this project, and Dr. Deb Margolis for supporting this endeavor.

Thank you Dr. Richard Ayers and Dr. Russ Olwell for your unwavering patience and expert guidance as I navigated the details of the findings. Your support and helpful insights were invaluable.

A special heartfelt appreciation to my exceptional editor, Dr. Sheryl Howie, whose meticulous proofreading and suggestions significantly enhanced the readability and flow of the text. I appreciate the attention to detail and knowledge of the intricacies of APA 7th edition.

Additionally, a thank you to the entire editorial and publishing team at Routledge. Your collective efforts, dedication, and professionalism have been indispensable in completing this project.

Lastly, and most importantly, I want to express my deepest gratitude, appreciation, and love to my family. Your support, patience, understanding, and encouragement kept me going. Your presence throughout this project has been a great source of motivation.

1 Introduction and Book Structure

> My students could not tell you what an aquarium is but can explain the process to boot up heroin.
>
> – Sadie, Second-Grade Teacher, New Hampshire

In the hallways of American schools, a silent crisis unfolds. Our schools are in the trenches, enduring the complexities of the opioid epidemic while navigating childhood trauma and adverse childhood experiences associated with students' exposure to community and household opioid-substance abuse. Educators share the untold stories of young children struggling with the extensive consequences of their exposure to the opioid crisis and the inadvertent impacts on the classroom and schools. This comprehensive exploration reveals the profound influence of the crisis on schools, exposing the emotional and professional impacts on educators while also enduring a global pandemic that only intensifies an already-intricate web of challenges.

The results of this multiple-case-study investigation, and two follow-up qualitative studies, create an in-depth understanding of the complexity of the opioid epidemic's influence schools in opioid-crisis regions. Through multiple points of data collection, follow-up investigations, and voices of educators working from the front lines, this is not just a story of crisis; the findings of this study generate a call to action for comprehensive, collaborative solutions that exceed the boundaries of the classroom and incorporate collective efforts from all stakeholders in the fight for the future of education in the United States.

Background and Context

The opioid epidemic in the United States has continued to develop into a complex crisis, leaving lasting impacts on communities, families, and individuals. This research is an exploration study of the complex consequences of the opioid epidemic on education, focusing on diverse aspects such as its

DOI: 10.4324/9781003378204-1

history, trends, data collected, documents, and implications for students, educators, and schools. The study investigates the critical challenges of childhood trauma and adverse childhood experiences (ACEs) within the context of opioid exposure and its impact on schools. Using multiple case studies to create a deep understanding of the phenomenon, the research uncovers the impact of the opioid epidemic on three schools in crisis regions. It offers insights into the experiences and highlights the voices of educators, shedding light on the emotional and professional impact of the opioid epidemic in schools.

Furthermore, a follow-up study, revisiting participants four years later, exposed the impact the pandemic and related school closures had on schools already coping with the opioid crisis, demonstrating intensified challenges faced by school districts, educators, and students. A third study is also shared to support external validity to generalize findings. In collaboration with all findings, the research uncovered district needs and potential interventions and strategies to address the complex issues surfacing from the consequences of the opioid epidemic in schools.

The needed interventions advocate for a comprehensive, multi-tiered approach involving collaboration among various stakeholders. Through a synthesis of multiple case studies, two additional qualitative follow-up investigations, and the voices of educators working on the front lines, the combined research provides a comprehensive understanding of the interconnected challenges posed by the opioid epidemic on education in the United States.

Statement of the Problem

The opioid epidemic was declared a public health emergency in 2017, and it continues to have a long and troubling trajectory across the United States, profoundly affecting not only individuals and families but also communities and schools. The statistics are concerning, with over 932,000 lives lost to drug overdoses from 1999 to 2021, and nearly 75% of drug overdose deaths in 2020 involving opioids (Hedegaard et al., 2015; WONDER, 2021). The gravity of this situation cannot be overstated, and despite the declaration of a public health emergency, the number of opioid-related deaths continues to rise, reaching 80,411 reported overdose deaths in 2021 as compared to 68,630 in 2020 (WONDER, 2023).

As the epidemic continues, schools find themselves on the front lines of this crisis, dealing with the far-reaching consequences beyond immediate health concerns. Children born into families coping with the consequences of opioid misuse face adversities that can manifest as social, emotional, and cognitive disabilities, impacting their ability to learn, engage, and thrive in school (Crouch, 2019; Drescher et al., 2022; Herranz et al., 2014; Jimenez et al., 2016; Nunes et al., 2015; Peisch et al., 2018).

The opioid epidemic is reshaping the educational landscape in many locations across the country, with children born with Neonatal Abstinence Syndrome (NAS) or into households battling addiction and facing unique challenges. Studies reveal a direct link between prenatal opioid exposure and developmental issues such as cognitive deficits, language weaknesses, and attention disorders, necessitating early interventions and specialized support services once these children enter school (Beckwith & Burke, 2015; Fill et al., 2018; McGlone & Mactier, 2015; Ornoy et al., 2010; Yuan et al., 2014).

While the opioid epidemic has prompted various state and community initiatives, the empirical literature on its direct educational impact remains limited. Policies addressing the crisis primarily stem from the health and community sector, with a recent emphasis on state-level initiatives to support education and prevention efforts. Programs like Narcan availability in schools, increased drug education, and trauma-informed care are steps in the right direction (SAMHSA, 2018). However, as the results of this study specify, more targeted efforts are needed to address the specific needs of students, educators, and schools impacted by the opioid epidemic. The findings and trends make it clear that as the crisis continues to evolve, so must our response.

Objectives of the Study

This research study is a comprehensive exploration of the educational impact of the opioid epidemic in the United States, particularly on elementary schools in crisis regions of the Northeastern United States. Through the lens of the schools and perspectives of the educators, the purpose of the study was to understand how the opioid epidemic affects students, educators, and schools, with a specific focus on the intersection of adverse childhood experiences, opioid exposure, and educational challenges. Additionally, the study investigated the preparedness of schools, the unfolding impact on special education, and the layers of support needed.

The study further extended its investigation by conducting a follow-up study to examine the effects of the COVID-19 pandemic on schools in opioid-crisis regions, providing a more comprehensive understanding of the ongoing challenges. A third investigation into external schools in other districts was also conducted to see if the results were specific to the case-study locations or if there was external validity to generalize impact across geographical locations.

The objective was to uncover and document the impact of the opioid epidemic on schools to better understand and comprehend the phenomenon. As the study unfolded, it was evident that the results contributed to a need for further investigations, which include collaborative, systemic interventions involving policymakers, educators, and communities to create strong communities for students and educators in schools struggling with the consequences of the opioid epidemic.

Research Questions

The study was a comprehensive exploration to better understand the educational impact of the opioid epidemic on elementary schools in crisis regions of the Northeastern United States by answering the following research questions:

1. How is the opioid epidemic impacting elementary schools in opioid-crisis regions of the Northeast?
2. How are schools located in opioid-crisis regions proactively preparing for the influx of students affected by the opioid epidemic entering the school?
3. How are schools in opioid-crisis regions developing and implementing professional development for administrators, teachers, and school staff to address the needs of students impacted by the opioid crisis?

The research questions are answered throughout the book, and many unintentional findings are shared to create a more comprehensive overall understanding of this ongoing public health emergency as it applies to schools and education.

The aim was to understand the complex and extensive ways the opioid epidemic impacts students, teachers, and schools. The goal was to contribute valuable insights that inform evidence-based policies and practices and to create a foundation for further studies and investigations of proposed interventions.

Significance of the Study

The research focused on the educational implications of the opioid epidemic, which is of paramount importance as it addresses a critical public health crisis and contributes to the existing body of knowledge in the field of education. This study went beyond the immediate health concerns associated with opioid use and explored the complicated and profound impact this crisis has on students, teachers, and schools.

One key aspect that emphasizes the significance of this research is its holistic approach to understanding challenges through the perspectives and lens of the educators working in the field every day. By examining the effects of ACEs, trauma, and unmet basic needs on students' ability to learn and educators' capacity to teach effectively, the study provided a comprehensive view of the complex issues faced by schools in opioid-crisis regions.

Methodology Preview

The study employed a multiple-case-study design to reveal patterns and themes across selected schools, shedding light on the implications of the opioid crisis on education and following Yin's (2018) definition of case study as an empirical method investigating contemporary phenomena within real-world contexts. This approach sought convergence in triangulating evidence to identify consistent patterns and themes in schools located in opioid-crisis regions. The study targeted public schools in opioid-crisis regions of Massachusetts, New Hampshire, and Maine. Three school districts were chosen based on significantly elevated overdose rates. Surveys and interviews included administrators, special education professionals, and kindergarten through second-grade teachers, ensuring a comprehensive understanding of the issue from various perspectives. Data collection incorporated surveys, interviews, the analysis of documents, the gathering of professional development plans, and archival information. The analysis employed in vivo, descriptive, and pattern coding to identify overarching themes and patterns across the selected cases (Saldana, 2016). Triangulation of data sources and member checking enhanced the credibility of the findings, providing a more comprehensive understanding of the phenomenon. An audit trail and a field journal were maintained to track steps and minimize biases.

Ethical Considerations

The research maintained ethical standards by ensuring the confidentiality of participants and school districts. All participations were voluntary and required informed consent. Participants were protected with anonymity and confidentiality, confirming no potential for harm. The school names were changed, and the participants' names were not released in the study. Pseudonyms are given to all participants in the field journal and named quotes. All necessary steps were taken to protect the rights and welfare of participants in all three studies discussed in this book. The three separate studies within this one overarching study were all approved through appropriate Internal Review Boards (IRBs), validating the adherence to ethical guidelines.

Organizational Structure of the Book – Chapter Overviews

This book is divided into three parts, comprising 14 chapters. Part 1 (Chapters 2–5) serves as the foundational part, offering insights into the research methodology and the opioid epidemic. It explores the historical context, legislative responses, prevailing trends, and the implications for students, educators, and schools.

Part 2 (Chapters 6–10) shares findings from educators' perspectives, as expressed through their voices and lenses. This part also incorporates entries from the field journal at the beginning of each chapter to share stories and experiences engaging in research in the field at the schools.

Part 3 (Chapters 11–14) explores the data and findings, explains extension studies, discusses relevant theories and nationwide educational trends, explores interventions, and outlines potential areas for future research.

What follows is an overview of each part and chapter of this book.

Part 1

The opioid epidemic in the United States has emerged as a complex crisis, continuing to create evolving impacts on communities, families, and individuals. Part 1 of the book, Chapters 2–5, lays the foundation and explores the consequences of the opioid epidemic on education, focusing on diverse aspects such as its historical roots, transitional trends in drug use, and the implications for students and schools. It further shares critical challenges posed by NAS and ACEs within the context of opioid exposure and educational implications. Part 1 also explores the research methodology and introduces the school district and educators participating.

Chapter 2

Schools are not immune to the consequences of the opioid epidemic. Chapter 2 shares a historical understanding of where we are now, how we got here, and the educational impact of the opioid crisis based on research available, associated policy, and publicly available data.

The opioid epidemic in the United States constitutes a profound crisis, claiming over 932,000 lives since 1999 (WONDER, 2023). Despite former president Donald Trump declaring it a public health emergency in 2017, opioid-related overdoses continued to rise. The epidemic originated from the overprescribing of opioids, leading to legislative attempts to address the overprescribing that inadvertently fueled heroin use (Haffajee & Mello, 2017). The crisis evolved to synthetic opioids like Fentanyl, which accounted for 88% of opioid-related deaths in 2021 (Centers for Disease Control and Prevention, National Center for Injury Prevention and Control, 2023). This chapter discusses the impact on children born into affected families, who face adverse childhood experiences and developmental challenges, which then poses a significant challenge for schools due to a surge in NAS and ACEs. Schools and educators are now tasked with addressing the educational and social-emotional needs of students impacted. Educational policies are evolving to incorporate prevention initiatives, including Narcan administration and relevant curricula. State programs and community initiatives are shared to emphasize the multifaceted responses. In summary, the opioid epidemic has created an educational crisis necessitating comprehensive responses, and Chapter 2 emphasizes the importance of further research to understand its full impact on education in schools in crisis regions.

Chapter 3

Chapter 3 explores the link between ACEs and the opioid epidemic's impact on children. ACEs, which encompass traumatic events, are often evident in families and communities impacted by substance use, heightening the risk of maltreatment, abuse, and challenging family dynamics. The ACE Pyramid illustrates how these experiences disrupt neurodevelopment, contributing to potential social, emotional, cognitive, and health impairments (CDC, 2014 & Felitti et al., 2019). Such impairments would require school interventions emphasizing the connection between ACEs, family opioid addiction, and academic struggles. Specifically, according to Kaiser Permanente Thriving Schools (n.d), children with three or more ACEs are five times more likely to have attendance issues, six times more likely to have behavior problems, and three times more likely to experience academic failure. When a person experiences frequent, intense, or prolonged adversity, such as caregiver's substance abuse, exposure to violence, chronic neglect, or physical or emotional abuse, it can result in profound adverse effects on the mind and body that can impact health and learning (Harvard University's Center for the Developing Child, 2022).

Chapter 3 contends that the ongoing opioid crisis poses far-reaching societal consequences, particularly affecting children. The ACE study serves as a crucial theoretical framework for understanding the broader implications of the opioid crisis on students and schools in affected communities.

Chapter 4

Chapter 4 shares the research methodology used to explore the impact of the opioid epidemic on elementary schools located in crisis regions of the Northeastern United States. Using Yin's (2018) multiple-case -study design, three schools in Massachusetts, New Hampshire, and Maine were investigated to understand how the opioid epidemic impacts the schools and how the schools prepared for and supported students directly impacted. Data collection involved surveys, interviews, publicly available data collection, and document analysis, with participants including educators, counselors, support staff, and administrators in public schools within opioid-crisis regions. The analysis utilized three rounds of coding: vivo coding, descriptive coding, and pattern coding (Saldana, 2016), which was supported by data triangulation, member checking, and an audit trail for validity (Creswell & Creswell, 2018). The study aimed to understand educators' experiences, comprehend student impact, uncover district preparedness, and discover the district's professional development plans in addressing the needs of students impacted by the opioid crisis.

Chapter 5

Chapter 5 shares background information on the participants and the schools investigated. With a total of 76 educators, the study's stringent selection criteria were based on CDC data and community law enforcement data identifying regions with opioid overdose rates exceeding the national average. Participants, including administrators, teachers, support staff, and social workers, exhibited diverse experience levels, ranging from under 5 to over 20 years in the field. The Massachusetts Anderson Loop School, New Hampshire Cobbs Hill School, and Maine Fox Hollow United School shared similarities in size, socioeconomic status, and concerns about the epidemic's impact, despite geographical differences. With participation rates ranging from 63% to 74% of the total number of qualified educators, the study captures a collection of knowledge and experiences of the crisis through different perspectives.

Part 2

The opioid crisis creates a complex atmosphere, profoundly impacting students, schools, and educators. In Part 2, educators' stories are shared to better understand the experiences, heartaches, and perspectives of those working in schools located in opioid epicenters. The stories vividly portray teachers' emotional strain and unwavering dedication amid the challenging landscape. Part 2 of the book includes Chapters 6–10. It explores the daunting student challenges educators face, such as exposure to countless adverse childhood experiences, homelessness, transiency, inadequate responses from the Department of Youth Services, and parental instability, among others. Despite initiatives by school districts, teachers expressed a sense of unpreparedness in their schools, emphasizing the lack of professional development and resources. This part highlights impactful quotes and unforgettable stories of our devoted educators working in crisis areas. Part 2 also shares entries from the field journals to create an additional understanding of experiences and observations while on location.

Chapter 6

Chapter 6 explores the far-reaching consequences of the opioid epidemic on schools in New Hampshire, Maine, and Massachusetts. In Cobbs Hill School and Fox Hollow United School, students grappled with exposure to drug-related behaviors and parental instability, fostering an environment where teachers are concerned about the normalization of drug culture and the trauma students experienced witnessing overdoses and other drug-related activities and crimes. The Anderson Loop School in Massachusetts faced similar challenges, with educators expressing worries about environmental factors like family drug use, poverty, homelessness, and parental instability affecting students. In all three schools, parental instability contributed to student stress, affecting well-being and focus, prompting concerns about day-to-day school operations. Survey results indicated that a high number of students were removed from their homes due to household addiction and exposure to serious crimes. Opioid exposure emerged within 100% ($N = 29$) of the participants who were interviewed. Other central themes associated with exposure that emerged in the interviews were student behaviors 100% ($N = 29$) and parent and family instability 100% ($N = 29$). Also notable that emerged in collected survey data, educators report the following situations stem from opioid exposure were child neglect 93% ($n = 62$), family instability 87% ($n = 58$), and involvement with the Department of Youth Services 79% ($n = 53$). Teachers shared their stories, and impactful quotes are highlighted throughout the chapter. Overall, the opioid crisis creates a complex atmosphere impacting students, families, and educators.

Chapter 7

In Chapter 7, student attendance circumstances associated with the opioid epidemic created a cycle of challenges for students, schools, and academic services. The findings revealed that homelessness, transiency, poverty, and living instability stemming from household addiction significantly disrupt classrooms. Educators shared stories and attributed these challenges to the root cause of addiction. The instabilities are negatively impacting students' academic progress and routines. Interviews and surveys stress the prevalence of transiency and homelessness as major factors affecting classrooms. Based on an analysis of the 29 interviews, 28 out of the 29 educators mentioned transiency and homelessness as significantly impacting the classroom or the school. Additionally, in the 67-participant surveys, 57 participants experienced a situation that resulted in a student's removal from the home because of a drug-related situation, 58 participants had students living with a relative because of household addiction, and 45 survey participants had students with open cases with the departments of youth services. In combination, 87% ($n = 58$) of all survey participants experienced the challenges of living in a home with active addiction that impacted attendance and the day-to-day operations of the school. Across all three schools, attendance teams and initiatives worked to address these issues.

Chapter 8

Chapter 8 illuminates the profound repercussions of the opioid crisis on educators. Based on an analysis of the 29 interviews, 79% mentioned scenarios and feelings that would be considered secondary trauma. Teachers coping with a continuously escalating epidemic found themselves burdened not only with the traditional role of the teacher but also with addressing students' basic needs stemming from the crisis. An unanticipated yet prominent theme that developed in the study was secondary educator trauma. Students' needs, neglect, and pain impact teachers, as shared through the quotes of the educators. Interviews and surveys uncovered teachers facing nontraditional expectations, contending with students traumatized by neglect and abuse, and exposure to crime. The emotional toll is palpable, leading to reported instances of secondary trauma, exhaustion, and even medical leave required due to post-traumatic stress disorder and panic attacks among teachers. Despite facing challenges, educators displayed remarkable compassion, extending their roles to provide essential student support. However, this continuous exposure to trauma takes a toll on teachers' mental well-being. Chapter 8 vividly portrays the emotional strain and unwavering dedication of teachers amid the challenging landscape of the opioid epidemic.

Chapter 9

Chapter 9 explores the profound impact of the opioid crisis on education, emphasizing the daunting challenges faced by educators in addressing the diverse needs of affected students. It reveals a surge in students requiring interventions and possibly special education services, showcasing educators' concerns about their readiness to tackle associated issues such as trauma and mental health disorders. Chapter 9 exposes a significant gap in educator's professional development and understanding of associated disabilities. Since the weight of the interventions was on the teachers, teachers admitted to feeling unprepared to address the needs of the students exposed to the epidemic or born with challenges associated with NAS. In fact, only 8% reported having any training working with students exposed to the epidemic, and only 21% reported feeling prepared to teach the students impacted by challenges and disabilities associated with opioid exposure. Despite initiatives by school districts, teachers expressed a sense of unpreparedness, emphasizing the lack of professional development and resources. The study highlights educators' concerns about the strain on resources and its prevalent impact on students' well-being.

Chapter 10

Chapter 10 uncovers documented attempts, both successful and unsuccessful, to fulfill some of the districts' needs regarding the opioid epidemic.

Although a mere 21% of educators felt adequately equipped to assist students grappling with challenges linked to the epidemic, the study revealed diverse approaches among districts in supporting affected students. In Maine's Fox Hollow, a focus on mental health and equality was evident, with the appointment of a director of clinical and behavior supports and a social-emotional learning (SEL) coach. Massachusetts' Anderson Loop School employed a truant/attendance officer to combat chronic absenteeism. Meanwhile, New Hampshire's Cobbs Hill School implemented mental health services, a resilience curriculum, and a trauma consultant for a trauma-sensitive environment. Reoccurring solutions in all three schools were free medical and dental evaluations, food and weather-appropriate clothing provided at no cost, and before- and after-school programs that provided a safe place to stay before and after school.

Though not explicitly credited for aiding children impacted by the opioid epidemic, these initiatives benefitted all children. The chapter concludes by identifying needs that arose in the research across the three schools, for example, emphasizing the importance of additional staff, mental health providers, social workers, and professional development on opioid crisis-related issues. Funding and community resources are crucial for effective solutions addressing the multifaceted challenges of the epidemic in schools.

Part 3

Part 3 (Chapters 11–14) consists of two post-pandemic research studies, one as a follow-up with the original case-study participants and the other to prove external validity. The chapters in Part 3 reveal the complex interplay between the opioid epidemic, students, teachers, schools, district leadership, and society. The discussion explores the connections to theories, literature, and current national education trends. By linking its findings to national issues such as teacher attrition, chronic absenteeism, and the broader teacher shortage, the study positions its findings within the larger educational landscape. Equally important is that the research findings highlighted in Part 3 of this book contribute to proposing practical interventions and solutions for further investigations and offer actionable steps to address the challenges identified. Part 3 highlights the potential to inform education policies and practices, especially in regions impacted by the opioid epidemic.

Chapter 11

Chapter 11 provides a concise and informative analysis, highlighting the profound impact of the opioid epidemic on schools in crisis regions, encompassing environmental, community, and household exposures. Adverse experiences, trauma, poverty, and homelessness directly affected teachers, attendance, budgets, preparation, special education services, administrative initiatives, curriculum, student behaviors, and the school's role in meeting basic needs. Through detailed tables summarizing interview themes, survey results, and reported student behaviors, the chapter emphasizes the multifaceted repercussions. Noteworthy findings included key themes prevalent in over 50% of the 29 interviews, calibrated survey outcomes across three case studies, and insights into educator preparedness and professional development opportunities. The research showcases the epidemic's direct influence on schools and the allocated preparedness by school districts for this public health emergency.

Aligning with existing literature on developmental challenges in households affected by substance abuse, a visual representation emphasizing the interconnectedness of environmental factors, ACEs, and community influences on schools. The chapter advocates for proactive preparation and support for educators navigating the complex challenges posed by the opioid epidemic.

Chapter 12

Chapter 12 presents a follow-up study revisiting the three case-study locations four years later in 2023, building on the 2018–2019 investigation. Examining the intersection of the opioid epidemic and the aftermath of the pandemic's impact, the research highlighted challenges faced by schools. Public health emergencies, such as the COVID-19 pandemic, contribute to disparities linked to child maltreatment risk factors (Conrad-Hiebner & Byram, 2020; Wong et al., 2021), compounding the existing challenges of the opioid epidemic. Seventeen educators from the original study share updates. Of those 17 participants, 13 agreed to an interview. Results indicate that challenges from the COVID-19 pandemic amplified trauma, attendance, food insecurity, secondary teacher trauma, and transiency challenges. One hundred percent mentioned challenges with the response of the Department of Youth Services. There are some notable mentions: all three locations show an increase in chronic absenteeism mentioned by 100% of participants, 69% mentioned leadership turnover, and 69% mentioned teacher shortages. Despite some new initiatives, post-pandemic challenges are more complex and pertinent in opioid-crisis regions.

Themes mirrored the original study; a follow-up study confirmed validity. The impact of the opioid crisis on schools and educators applies broadly across different geographic locations.

Chapter 13

Chapter 13 delves into the intricate challenges faced by schools in areas affected by the opioid epidemic, emphasizing the convergence of ACEs and Maslow's hierarchy of needs. Highlighting the profound impact of unmet basic needs, trauma, and adverse experiences on students' learning capabilities and teachers' effectiveness, the discussion draws on Maslow's theory to underscore the pivotal role of fulfilling fundamental needs for academic growth. The opioid crisis and related ACEs exacerbated these challenges, leading to heightened stress, mental health issues, and unmet needs for students. Additionally, the chapter explores the alarming link between teacher stress, secondary trauma, and the opioid crisis, contributing to a national trend of high teacher turnover and dissatisfaction. Another national crisis, post-pandemic chronic absenteeism influenced by ACEs, is worsened by the opioid crisis.

Chapter 14

Schools and communities located in opioid-crisis regions serve as catalysts for transformative change. Acknowledging the profound understanding of students' daily realities, where trauma and adverse childhood experiences often overshadow learning, educators become frontline responders, providing essential support beyond academics. However, the toll on educators' mental and student needs demands attention and systemic support. This chapter presents 18 interventions, from targeted professional development to a multi-sectoral approach, offering suggestions for further explorations and research focusing on solutions for schools to become resilient communities. By implementing these interventions, communities, policymakers, and educators can collaboratively pave the way for a brighter future, fostering a nurturing environment that addresses academic and mental health needs. This collective effort seeks to transform schools into resilient communities capable of navigating the complexities of the opioid crisis and other challenges faced by students today.

Personal Perspectives and Biases

In full transparency, I want to disclose that before entering higher education, I spent over a decade as a special education teacher in two school districts situated in regions coping with the potential of becoming an opioid crisis district. One of those districts was not just my workplace but also my hometown, where I witnessed firsthand the devastating impact of the opioid epidemic on the lives of friends, colleagues, and families. I established connections with those affected within the school district and community. I had friends, classmates, and acquaintances that I grew up with who overdosed or are still coping with their opioid-use disorder and addictions. Many times, the addiction stemmed from a sports injury or a root canal along with a prescription for a pain killer. I grew up in the gray period, when opioids were not supposed to be addictive, according to the marketing campaigns.

Then, around 2015–2016, as an educator in a community school, I observed the transformation of the school, shifts in family structures with more grandparents assuming caregiving roles, more Department of Youth Services open cases, increased opioid overdoses, and a noticeable rise in childhood traumas. Through further conversations with families, colleagues, and children, it was shared that there were household and environmental exposures to opioid-use disorders and associated substance abuse.

During that period, before 2017, the prioritization of resources, mental health support, and interventions for such issues was lagging. This gap encouraged me to explore this research to understand and fully comprehend the phenomenon more deeply.

Although this research project did not directly involve my community, given my experience, monitoring and acknowledging biases were essential. I maintained a detailed field journal, documenting notes, memoranda, and an audit trail that transparently outlined the research process, from project initiation to developing and reporting findings. This journal served as a tool to separate personal thoughts from facts and findings, continuously tracking and bracketing biases.

Considering my past experiences, community involvement, the extended time I spent at each research location, and the inherent nature of the research, tracking and bracketing through a field journal became necessary to minimize biases and increase objectivity. Some of my perspectives and journal entries, sharing personal experiences, were incorporated into this book to help explain the impacts of the phenomenon.

Key Terms

Adverse childhood experiences (ACEs) are potentially traumatic events that occur in childhood (0–17 years) (CDC, 2014).

The Department of Youth Services (DYS) is the juvenile justice and child protection agency in Massachusetts. Their mission is to make communities safer by improving outcomes for youth (Department of Youth Services, 2023).

Note: Different states referred to their child protection agency with different titles. Participants from the study typically used acronyms such as DYS, DCF, DHHS, and DCYF. Generally speaking, the agency is referred to as DYS in the text (regardless of location except in verbatim quotes) to keep it consistent throughout the book.

Neonatal Abstinence Syndrome (NAS) is a term used when babies are exposed to drugs in the womb before birth. Babies can then go through drug withdrawal after birth. The syndrome most often applies to opioid medicines (Boston's Children's Hospital, n.d.).

Neonatal Opioid Withdrawal Syndrome (NOWS) is a term used when babies are exposed to opioids in the womb before birth. Babies can then go through drug withdrawal after birth (Weller et al., 2021).

Note: Most literature refers to NAS even when referring to opioid exposure. Within the chapters, although NOWS is introduced, NAS is the term used when referring to prenatal opioid exposure.

Opioids are a class of drugs that include the illegal drug heroin, synthetic opioids such as fentanyl, and pain relievers available legally by prescription, such as oxycodone (OxyContin®), hydrocodone (Vicodin®), codeine, morphine, and many others (NIDA, 2023).

The McKinney-Vento Homeless Assistance Act: The McKinney-Vento Homeless Assistance Act is a U.S. federal law that provides money for homeless shelter programs. Subtitle VII-B of The McKinney-Vento Homeless Assistance Act authorizes the federal Education for Homeless Children and Youth (EHCY) Program and is federal legislation related to the education of children experiencing homelessness (NCHE, 2023).

Acknowledgments of Special Permissions

Permission was granted to reprint materials in this book by different organizations, publishing companies, and non-profits. I want to acknowledge the following groups and individuals for special permission to reprint and for the use of materials.

EdWeek Research Center, in collaboration with Merrimack College Winston School of Education and Social Policy (2023), for permission to use and publish graphs, tables, and visuals from the 2023 Merrimack College National Teacher Survey.

Attendance Works, a national nonprofit, and the Everyone Graduates Center at John Hopkins University (2023), for the analysis of data (and permissions to recreate an associated graph) released by the U.S. Department of Education for the 2018–2019 and 2021–2022 school years.

Phi Delta Kappan for permission and released copyright to use quotes throughout this book originally published in Welby, K. A. (2019a). Coping with the opioid crisis: Teachers need support right now. *Phi Delta Kappan*, *101*(3), 53–56.

The ToolBox Project (n.d.) for allowing me the privilege of highlighting the Tool Box Poster Visual within this book.

I want to acknowledge that a portion of this project was completed in part of my doctoral dissertation, *The Implications of the Opioid Epidemic on Select Elementary Schools in Crisis Regions of the Northeast: A Multiple Case Study Investigation* (2019b).

References

Beckwith, A. M., & Burke, S. A. (2015). Identification of early developmental deficits in infants with prenatal heroin, methadone, and other opioid exposure. *Clinical Pediatrics, 54*(4), 328.

Boston's Children's Hospital. (n.d.). https://www.childrenshospital.org/conditions/neonatal-abstinence-syndrome-nas

Center for the Developing Child. (2022). *Toxic stress.* Harvard University. https://developingchild.harvard.edu/science/key-concepts/toxic-stress/#:~:text=Toxic%20stress%20response%20can%20occur,hardship%E2%80%94without%20adequate%20adult%20support

Centers for Disease Control and Prevention, National Center for Injury Prevention and Control. (2023). *Drug overdose deaths.* https://www.cdc.gov/drugoverdose/deaths/index.html

Centers for Disease Control and Prevention. (2014). *The ACE pyramid.* National Center for Injury Prevention and Control, Division of Violence Prevention. https://www.cdc.gov/violenceprevention/acestudy/about.html

Conrad-Hiebner, A., & Byram, E. (2020). The temporal impact of economic insecurity on child maltreatment: A systematic review. *Trauma, Violence, & Abuse, 21*(1), 157–178. https://doi.org/10.1177/1524838018756122

Creswell, J. W., & Creswell, J. D. (2018). *Research design: Qualitative, quantitative, and mixed methods approaches* (5th ed.). SAGE.

Crouch, E., Radcliff, E., Hung, P., & Bennett, K. (2019). Challenges to school success and the role of adverse childhood experiences. *Academic Pediatrics, 19*(8), 899–907. https://doi-org.proxy3.noblenet.org/10.1016/j.acap.2019.08.006

Department of Youth Services. (2023). *As the Juvenile Justice agency for the Commonwealth of Massachusetts, the Department of Youth Services promotes positive change in the youth in our care and custody.* https://www.mass.gov/orgs/department-of-youth-services

Drescher, J., Steyer, L., Townley-Flores, C., & Humphreys, K. (2022). Has the opioid crisis affected student learning? A national analysis of growth rates. *The ANNALS of the American Academy of Political and Social Science, 703*(1), 234–261. https://doi.org/10.1177/00027162231151524

Everyone Graduates Center at John Hopkins University. (2023). *Rising tide of chronic absence challenges schools.* https://new.every1graduates.org/

Felitti, V. J., Anda, R. F., Nordenberg, D., Williamson, D. F., Spitz, A. M., Edwards, V., Koss, M. P., & Marks, J. S. (2019). Relationship of childhood abuse and household dysfunction to many of the leading causes of death in adults: The adverse childhood experiences (ACE) study (reprint). *American Journal of Preventive Medicine, 56*(6), 774–786. https://doi-org.proxy3.noblenet.org/10.1016/j.amepre.2019.04.001

Fill, M. A., Miller, A. M., Wilkinson, R. H., Warren, M. D., Dunn, J. R., Schaffner, W., & Jones, T. F. (2018). Educational disabilities among children born with neonatal abstinence syndrome. *Pediatrics, 152*(3), 1–8. https://doi.org/10.1542/peds.2018-0562

Haffajee, R. L., & Mello, M. M. (2017). Drug companies' liability for the opioid epidemic. *The New England Journal of Medicine, 377*(24), 2301–2305. https://doi.org/10.1056/NEJMp1710756

Hedegaard, H., Chen, L.-H., & Warner, M. (2015). Drug-poisoning deaths involving heroin: United States, 2000–2013. *NCHS Data Brief, 190*, 1–8.

Herranz, G. S., Vílchez, M. A. L., Ledo, J. D., & Sierra, A. M. (2014). Children born to heroin-addicted mothers: What's the outcome 25 years later? *Journal of Addiction Research and Therapy, 5*(180).

Jimenez, M. E., Wade, R., Jr., Lin, Y., Morrow, L. M., & Reichman, N. E. (2016). Adverse experiences in early childhood and kindergarten outcomes. *Pediatrics, 137*(2), e20151839.

Kaiser Permanente Thriving Schools (n.d). Adverse Childhood Expererienccs retrieved from: https://thrivingschools.kaiserpermanente.org/mental-health/aces/

McGlone, L., & Mactier, H. (2015). Infants of opioid-dependent mothers: Neurodevelopment at six months. *Early Human Development, 91*(1), 19–21.

Merrimack College Winston School of Education and Social Policy. (2023). *National teacher survey*. Education Week Research Center. https://www.merrimack.edu/academics/education-and-social-policy/about/merrimack-college-teacher-survey/

National Center for Homeless Education. (2023). https://nche.ed.gov/legislation/mckinney-vento/

National Institute for Drug Abuse. (2023). https://nida.nih.gov/research-topics/opioids

Nunes, E., Weissman, M., Goldsten, R., McAvay, G., Beckford, C., Seracini, A., & Wickramaratne, P. (2015). Psychiatric disorders and impairment in the children of opiate addicts: Prevalence and distribution by ethnicity. *American Journal on Addictions, 9*(3), 232–241.

Ornoy, A., Daka, L., Goldzweig, G., Gil, Y., Mjen, L., Levit, S., Shufman, E., Bar-Hamburger, R., & Greenbaum, C. (2010). Neurodevelopmental and psychological assessment of adolescents born to drug-addicted parents: Effects of SES and adoption. *Child Abuse & Neglect, 34*(5), 354–368.

Peisch, V., Sullivan, A. D., Breslend, N. L., Benoit, R., Sigmon, S. C., Forehand, G. L., Strolin-Goltzman, J., & Forehand, R. (2018). Parental opioid abuse: A review of child outcomes, parenting, and parenting interventions. *Journal of Child and Family Studies, 27*(7), 2082–2099. https://doi.org/10.1007/s10826-018-1061-0

Saldana, J. (2016). *The coding manual for qualitative researchers*. Sage Publications Inc.

Substance Abuse and Mental Health Services. (2018). *Opioid overdose prevention toolkit (HHS Publication No. SMA18-1472)*. U.S. Department of Health and Human Resources. https://store.samhsa.gov/system/files/sma18-4742.pdf

The ToolBox Project. (n.d.). *Tools for learning. Tools for life*. https://toolboxproject.com/

Welby, K. A. (2019a). Coping with the opioid crisis: Teachers need support right now. *Phi Delta Kappan, 101*(3), 53–56.

Welby, K. A. (2019b). *The implications of the opioid epidemic on select elementary schools in crisis regions of the Northeast: A multiple case study investigation*. Southern New Hampshire University.

Weller, A. E., Crist, R. C., Reiner, B. C., Doyle, G. A., & Berrettini, W. H. (2021). Neonatal opioid withdrawal syndrome (NOWS): A transgenerational echo of the opioid crisis. *Cold Spring Harbor Perspectives in Medicine, 11*(3), a039669. https://doi.org/10.1101/cshperspect.a039669

WONDER. (2021). *Wide-ranging online data for epidemiologic research Atlanta, GA: CDC*. Centers for Disease Control and Prevention. http://wonder.cdc.gov

WONDER. (2023). *Wide-ranging online data for epidemiologic research Atlanta, GA: CDC*. Centers for Disease Control and Prevention. http://wonder.cdc.gov

Wong, J. Y.-H., Wai, A. K.-C., Wang, M. P., Lee, J. J., Li, M., Kwok, J. Y.-Y., Wong, C. K.-H., & Choi, A. W-M. (2021). Impact of COVID-19 on child maltreatment: Income instability and parenting issues. *International Journal of Environmental Research and Public Health, 18*(4), 1501. http://dx.doi.org/10.3390/ijerph18041501

Yin, R. K. (2018). *Case study research and applications: Design and methods* (6th ed.). Sage.

Yuan, Q., Rubic, M., Seah, J., Rae, C., Wright, I. M., Kaltenbach, K., Feller, J. M., Abdel-Latif, M. E., Chu, C., & Oei, J. L. (2014). Do maternal opioids reduce neonatal regional brain volumes? A pilot study. *Journal of Perinatology, 34*(12), 909–913. https://doi.org/10.1038/jp.2014.111

Part 1

History, Participants, and Methodology

The opioid epidemic in the United States has emerged as a complex crisis, continuing to generate evolving impacts on communities, families, and individuals. Part 1 of the book, Chapters 2–5, lays the foundation and explores the consequences of the opioid epidemic on education, focusing on diverse aspects such as its historical roots, transitional trends in drug use, and the implications for students and schools. It further shares critical challenges posed by Neonatal Abstinence Syndrome (NAS) and adverse childhood experiences (ACEs) within the context of opioid exposure and educational implications. Part 1 also explores the research methodology and introduces the school district and the participating educators.

DOI: 10.4324/9781003378204-2

2 The Educational Impact of the Opioid Epidemic in the United States

> We have a huge number of students directly impacted by the epidemic here. Our kids know way too much. They know what different substances look like, they know street names, they have been held by gunpoint over a drug deal gone wrong, they have watched their parents and guardians inject heroin. They are taken out of their homes because of this epidemic. I would say that every single child in our school has experienced some type of trauma because of this epidemic. This impacts our school and my classroom.
>
> – Lucia, New Hampshire Special Education Teacher

Educators across the United States work in opioid epicenters surrounded by communities, families, and children impacted by addiction. An indirect consequence of the opioid epidemic is the positioning of educators in the battlefield fighting the impact of the crisis in educational settings across the country through attempts to provide students with what they need academically, socially, and emotionally, along with basic life requirements. The results of the epidemic continue to cause indirect harm to individuals, communities, and now schools. The unspoken reality is that countless schools in the United States are ground zero in battling the intense war that this opioid epidemic has created. Educators and schools are experiencing extreme ramifications of this widespread societal challenge. Schools and children are not immune to the impact of this crisis, and abundant evidence confirms that adverse home and community factors are associated with lost learning opportunities, which is precisely what is happening in hard-hit areas. We are only beginning to understand the far-reaching indirect consequences of the opioid crisis.

This chapter provides an overview of the opioid epidemic, the declaration of a public health emergency, the history of abuse, the children impacted, and school and policy responses. Collectively, it is a snapshot of the understanding of where we are now and how we got here.

DOI: 10.4324/9781003378204-3

The History of the Opioid Epidemic

The opioid epidemic has greatly impacted communities across the United States. The addiction and abuse of opioids are global problems that profoundly affect communities, schools, neighborhoods, and families. The misuse of opioids also affects the health and social and economic well-being of all societies. More than 932,000 people have died since 1999 from a drug overdose (WONDER, 2021). Nearly 75% of drug overdose deaths in 2020 involved an opioid (Hedegaard et al., 2021). Children are born into families dealing with the ramifications of opioids and misuse. Sometimes, families are in crisis and are struggling to battle this devastating and debilitating disease of addiction while trying their best to raise their children within the family unit. Living in a household battling substance abuse or exposure to drugs in utero is considered an adverse childhood experience that can lead to social, emotional, and cognitive disabilities (Felitti et al., 2019; Peisch et al., 2018).

The opioid epidemic was declared a public health emergency in 2017. Since 2017, the epidemic has shown no improvement with a steady increase in opioid-related overdoses (National Center for Health Statistics, 2021).

Declaration of a Public Health Emergency

On October 26, 2017, former president Donald Trump declared the opioid epidemic a public health emergency, stating, "We are currently dealing with the worst drug crisis in American history. . . . It has just been so long in the making. Addressing it will require all of our efforts" (President Donald Trump, 2017).

As requested by the presidential administration in 2017, former Health and Human Services (HHS) Secretary Eric D. Hargan issued the following statement upon the announcement of a nationwide public health emergency regarding the opioid crisis:

> Today's declaration, coupled with the President's direction that executive agencies use all appropriate emergency authorities and other relevant authorities, is another decisive action the Trump Administration is taking in response to America's deadly opioid crisis. President Trump has made this national crisis a top priority since he took office in January, and we are proud to be leading this effort at HHS. His call to action today brings a new level of urgency to the comprehensive strategy HHS unveiled under President Trump, which empowers the real heroes of this fight: the communities on the frontlines of the epidemic.
>
> (United States Press Release, 2017)

The press release and history behind the declared public health emergency were results of information that, according to Seth et al. (2018), more than 140 Americans were dying daily from drug overdoses, and precisely 91 were dying per day from opioid use. Other statistics included 52,404 Americans died from drug overdoses in 2015, and approximately 64,000 died in 2016.

Declaring a nationwide public health emergency accelerated appointments of specialized personnel to address this emergency. The goal was to improve access to prevention, treatment, and recovery support services, increase the availability and distribution of Narcan and other overdose-reversing drugs, strengthen public health data collection and reporting, advance pain management practice, and improve research. There was no mention of school support in any of the targeted interventions.

All the above appointments were in place. However, national overdose deaths involving opioids continued to increase. The figure below shows the total number of U.S. overdose deaths involving any opioid from 1999 to 2021. Any opioid includes prescription opioids, heroin, and synthetic opioids other than methadone (such as fentanyl). According to this figure (Wonder, 2023), opioid-involved overdose deaths increased from 21,089 in 2010 to 47,600 in 2017 and continued steadily through 2019. This was followed by a significant increase in 2020, with 68,630 reported deaths, and again in 2021, with 80,411 reported overdose deaths.

Since former president Donald Trump and former Health and Human Service Secretary declared the opioid epidemic a public health emergency in 2017, the state of the epidemic has taken a turn for the worse with a sharp increase in opioid overdoses over the past six years.

How did we get here?

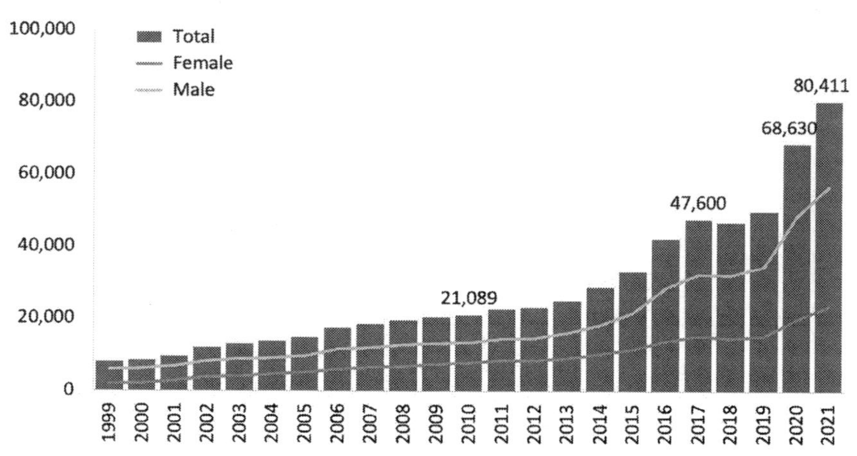

Figure 2.1 National overdose deaths involving any opioid, 1999–2021

Source: https://nida.nih.gov/research-topics/trends-statistics/overdose-death-rates

Opioid Abuse

The opioid epidemic appears to be initially rooted in the overprescribed number of opioids by healthcare professionals (Haffajee & Mello, 2017). According to the Centers for Disease Control and Prevention (2017), the United States is the largest opioid consumer globally. Research indicated that the majority of illicit users first misused prescription opioids. Tragically, this abuse continues to result in deaths, overdoses, and disruptions in communities and families nationwide.

Historically, the drastic increase in the number of prescribed opioids contributed to the severity of the current opioid epidemic nationwide. One may argue that the increased number of prescriptions written and dispensed and aggressive marketing by pharmaceutical companies have all contributed to the current opioid epidemic and abuse problem (Humphreys et al., 2022; Muhuri et al., 2013; Carlson et al., 2016). The number of prescriptions for opioids prescribed by healthcare providers increased drastically from 76 million in 1991 to nearly 259 million in 2012 – equivalent to one prescription for every adult in the United States (Paulozzi et al., 2014).

To help resolve the problem of increased numbers of prescriptions, state legislation has forced healthcare providers to limit prescriptions written for opiates. By 2018, more than 30 states considered 130 bills related to opioid prescribing habits. According to the National Conference of State Legislatures (NCSL, 2019), by December 2017, 24 states enacted legislation with some limits related to opioid prescribing. The temporary problem with this legislation, some might argue, is that limiting opioid prescriptions may result in increased heroin use. Individuals who are addicted need the medication, but efforts to limit opioid prescribing resulted in restricting prescriptions for opioids, and heroin became easier to obtain than opioids. Limited access to opioid prescriptions fueled heroin use. The availability and low cost of heroin in the United States were identified as significant contributors to rising rates of heroin use (DEA, 2015). Individuals are reportedly switching to heroin because it is cheaper and easier to obtain than prescription opioids. This evolving problem has led to a global crisis in transitioning from opioid pills to heroin and eventually to even more fatal synthetic opioids such as Fentanyl (National Institute on Drug Abuse [NIDA], 2021) and, most recently, Xylazine, a veterinary tranquilizer (Friedman et al., 2022). Heroin users start by using prescription opioid pain medications 80% of the time (Pollini et al., 2011). Heroin use and abuse increased across the United States regardless of sex, age group, and income level (CDC, 2017). Eventually, heroin was commonly laced with Fentanyl, a powerful synthetic opioid 50–100 times more potent than morphine. Synthetic opioids, including Fentanyl, are now the most common drug responsible for drug-related overdose deaths in the United States. In 2017, 59% of opioid-related deaths involved synthetic opioids, compared to 14% in 2010 (NIDA, 2021). Even

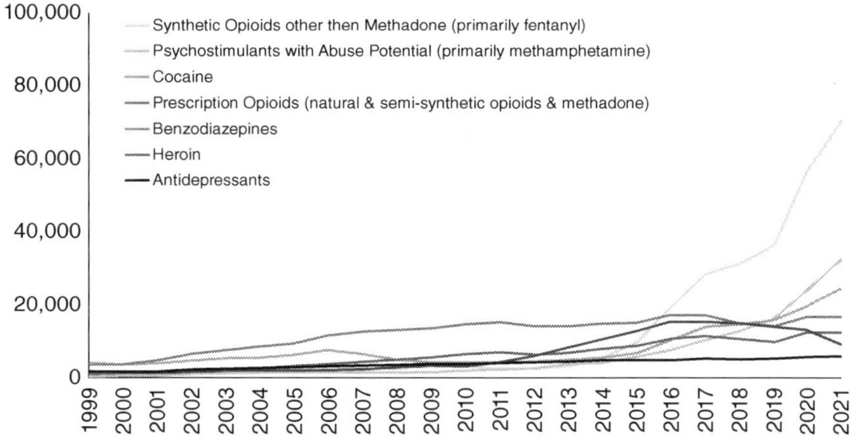

Figure 2.2 National drug overdose deaths number among all ages, 1999–2021

Source: https://nida.nih.gov/research-topics/trends-statistics/overdose-death-rates

more problematic, according to the National Center for Health Statistics (Ahmad et al., 2023), in 2020, 83.2% of opioid-related deaths involved a synthetic opioid. Deaths from overdose have evolved, starting with prescription opioids to heroin and eventually synthetic opioids, and that evolution continues to be more and more problematic.

Data from the National Institute on Drug Abuse (NIDA) (2021) show the dangerous trend of overdose deaths involving opioids. Figure 2.2 depicts the tragic increase in opioid abuse and deaths from 1999 to 2020 in the United States with a visual of the evolution of opioids from pills starting in 1999, leading to increased heroin deaths in 2011, followed by a sharp increase in synthetic opioid deaths starting in 2014–2015. The continued upward trend looks dire without intensive interventions.

The history of the opioid epidemic has resulted in many challenges in our society that need to be addressed. The societal challenges due to the epidemic will lead to continued and future ramifications in schools, neighborhoods, family structures, hospitals, and law enforcement agencies. These ramifications will be prominent in all communities for years. One of the complications is the increase in children born with Neonatal Abstinence Syndrome (NAS), Neonatal Opioid Withdrawal Syndrome (NOWS), or born into a household battling addiction.

The Children of the Opioid Epidemic

The opioid epidemic has direct and indirect implications for students in schools throughout the United States. Children are born suffering from opioid withdrawal at alarming rates across the country. Many of the students exposed to opioids in utero risk being born with a cognitive or language deficit (Beckwith & Burke, 2015; Fill et al., 2018; Kim et al., 2021; McGlone & Mactier, 2015; Nygaard et al., 2015; Ornoy et al., 2010; Yuan et al., 2014). The possibility of such disabilities could qualify children for early intervention services and special education services for academic and social-emotional needs once they enter school. Students who are living in the care of a parent or household with someone struggling with an opioid-use disorder may be at higher risk of experiencing trauma, school absences, social withdrawal, and behavior issues that can impact educational outcomes (Crouch, 2019; Drescher et al., 2022; Herranz et al., 2014; Jimenez et al., 2016; Nunes et al., 2015; Peisch et al., 2018). In addition to the direct link between parents and children, drug use in the community and exposure in the child's expanded social environment and network outside the home are also linked to negative consequences for the development and future of well-being children (Wolf et al., 2016). As the crisis continues to grow, more and more students are impacted and displaced from their homes. Many students are transient. Some are living with grandparents or entering foster care. These outcomes of the opioid epidemic impact children's ability to learn, engage, and thrive in school.

How did this happen?

Neonatal Abstinence Syndrome and Neonatal Opioid Withdrawal Syndrome

In the early 2010s, without the known ramifications of opioid abuse, women of childbearing age were prescribed opioid pain relievers by healthcare providers at an alarming rate. Prescription opioid overdose deaths among women have increased more than 400% from 1999 to 2010 and shortly after heroin overdose deaths among women have tripled (Hedegaard et al., 2015). A parallel trend with the increased number of opioid prescriptions was the aggressive marketing by pharmaceutical companies in the early 2000s (Muhuri et al., 2013; Carlson et al., 2016).

The upsurge of opioids prescribed to women led to many women suffering from addiction, misuse, and abuse of opioids (Hedegaard et al., 2015). Many women of childbearing age who were prescribed opioid pain relievers and became pregnant gave birth to infants who were dependent on opioids *in utero*. However, this was not the fault of the mothers and families. This began when the addictive properties of the prescribed pain medications were unknown to mothers who did not intend to put their children at risk. Nevertheless, many children were, and are still, born with NAS or NOWS (Hirai et al., 2021).

These scenarios are in addition to the generalized societal increase in overall opioid addiction.

Neonatal Abstinence Syndrome Statistics

NAS and NOWS occur when opioids pass through the placenta to the fetus during pregnancy. Exposure to opioids during pregnancy may lead the unborn baby to become dependent along with the mother. Some of the various short-term symptoms of NAS include excessive crying, seizures, fever, irritability, tremors, slow weight gain, diarrhea, vomiting, and possibly death. Long-term effects are cognitive, developmental, and behavioral disorders. NAS involves hospitalization and treatment with medication (often morphine) to relieve symptoms. Medication is slowly tapered off until the baby adjusts to being opioid-free. Many infants exposed to methadone during pregnancy typically also require treatment for NAS (O'Donnell et al., 2009).

The frequency of NAS in the United States doubled from 2009 to 2012 and has grown fivefold since 2000. NAS births have increased nationally by over 400% since 2000 (Winkelman et al., 2018). The swift rise in NAS parallels the upsurge in opioid use in the United States, especially among women of childbearing age. NAS is a rapidly growing public health problem that continues to grow (Jones, 2013).

Additionally, more recent data from the Healthcare Cost and Utilization Project (2021) stated that seven newborns are diagnosed with NAS for every 1,000 newborns in the hospital, with almost 80 diagnosed daily. Furthermore, the number of babies born with NAS in the United States increased by 82% from 2010 to 2017. Increases were reported in approximately all states and demographic groups (Hirai et al., 2021). According to the combination of data collection and available research, there appears to be a link between the number of opioid prescriptions per state and NAS per state (Patrick et al., 2015; Paulozzi et al., 2014).

Based on the research, it is expected that schools located in high-prescribing parts of the country, such as southeastern states and New England, are more likely to have the most significant educational challenges given the number of children entering the schools who live in a household with an increased probability of household addiction. Communities with a high number of NAS births will need to be more proactive, more aware, and more educated on the increased possibility of various challenges the schools and communities will face, and of the interventions needed to ensure these children have the tools and opportunities to succeed. To understand the necessary school interventions, there needs to be clarity on the developmental and social needs of children born with NAS.

Neonatal Abstinence Syndrome (NAS) and Development

Children born with NAS may experience developmental and cognitive challenges that should be addressed through infancy and beyond. According to research, prenatal opioid exposure could be associated with weaknesses in language, deficiencies in cognition, and attention/hyperactivity disorder (Beckwith & Burke, 2015; Lee et al., 2020; McGlone & Mactier, 2015; Nygaard et al., 2015; Ornoy et al., 2010; Yuan et al., 2014). These developmental challenges will most likely need interventions throughout the child's primary years and beyond.

Various studies and research indicate a link between NAS and cognitive and behavioral difficulties through infancy and beyond. There is much discussion on whether school-age children have academic and behavioral struggles because they were born with NAS or due to exposure to addiction.

The research into the developmental and cognitive impact of NAS is relatively new. Before 2010, there was limited research on whether prenatal exposure to opioids was linked to cognitive and behavioral disorders in children. Since 2010, with the increased prominence of the opioid addiction, additional studies were conducted on the development of children who were born exposed to opioids leading to NAS. Most research conducted since 2010 has concluded that there is a possible link between NAS and cognitive and behavioral disorders. Since 2010, a combination of research has found that the following are possible consequences of infants born with NAS: preterm birthweight and obstetric complications, respiratory insufficiency, heart defects, reduced growth, cognitive and motor ability deficits, attention-deficit hyperactivity disorder, lower IQ, behavioral problems, inattention, hyperactivity, and speech, language, and communication disorders. The combination of various studies provides adequate evidence that opioid exposure during pregnancy could result in developmental and cognitive deficiencies (Beckwith & Burke, 2015; McGlone & Mactier, 2015; Nygaard et al., 2015; Ornoy et al., 2010; Yuan et al., 2014). These challenges could qualify the children for special education services once the infant reaches school age.

Studies indicate that opioid exposure affects the regions that control neurocognitive processes such as attention, memory, motor speed, and visual-spatial processing. Specifically, Yuan et al. (2014) researched the brain functions and structures of infants at two maternity hospitals that were opioid exposed in utero. The brain scan results of babies born with NAS suggest that prenatal exposure to opioids may decrease the whole brain and basal ganglia volumes. These findings indicate that opioid exposure affects the regions that control neurocognitive processes such as attention, memory, motor speed, and visual-spatial processing (Yuan et al., 2015). A similar study by McGlone and Mactier (2015) found that infants with significant NAS are prone to a higher risk of developmental difficulties and delayed visual development. The study compares the neurodevelopment of 81 opioid-exposed infants to 50 children not born with NAS. The assessment administered in the study measures development trends that indicate intelligence and functional mental growth in children under two years old. The study concluded that at 6 months of age, infants born to methadone-maintained opioid-dependent mothers had lower developmental scores in all areas (locomotor, personal-social, language-hearing, eye-hand, and performance) than the infants who were not born exposed to opioids. These results also concluded that infants with significant NAS are at higher risk of developmental difficulties and delayed visual development (McGlone & Mactier, 2015).

Research conducted by Ornoy et al. (2010) focused on the neurodevelopmental and psychological assessment of adolescents born to drug-addicted mothers. This study examined the cognitive outcomes of babies born with NAS and investigated whether prenatal exposure to heroin may have long-term consequences for development during early and middle childhood. The research analyzed the cognitive, social, and emotional functioning of children exposed to drugs *in utero*. The results indicate that children exposed to at least one risk factor, such as exposure to drugs, low social and economic status, or adoption, performed worse than those not exposed to any of these risk factors. Drug exposure was also associated with adult ADHD-related problems (Ornoy et al., 2010). Furthermore, other research examined whether lower cognitive performances and behavior issues resulted from NAS or environmental factors. Research by Nygaard et al. (2015) explored the outcome of foster children born with NAS. The research focused on foster and adoptive children to determine if the children placed in a low-risk environment catch up cognitively. The research indicates that children exposed to opioids *in utero* did not catch up to peers over time. This is a consistent result even when the child is placed in a stable family at a very early age. Studies indicate there is an adverse effect of factors related to prenatal drug exposure to opioids over time (Nygaard et al., 2015).

These studies focused on the effects of prenatal opioid exposure in primary infancy and childhood. Results have shown that children prenatally exposed to opioids could show lower cognitive performance than non-exposed infants. Prenatal heroin and opioid exposure can be associated with language weaknesses, cognition deficiencies, and attention/hyperactivity disorder. Evidence also suggests that exposure to maternal opioids decreases brain volumes in newborn infants. This exposure contributes to the high occurrence of neurodevelopmental and behavioral problems seen in opioid-exposed children later in life (Beckwith & Burke, 2015; Fill et al., 2018; McGlone & Mactier, 2015; Nygaard et al., 2015; Ornoy et al., 2010; Yuan et al., 2014).

Dr. Margaret Fill et al. (2018) the Centers for Disease Control and Prevention (2017) conducted a longitudinal study in Tennessee that provided further evidence of the effects of opioid exposure in children and concluded that infants born with NAS are behind other children in school. Dr. Fill and colleagues followed infants born with NAS from birth to school age. Her study concluded that the children born with NAS were 44% more likely to be referred for an evaluation for developmental delays. Of the children born with NAS, 36% qualified in Tennessee for intervention and met the criteria for an educational disability.

Analysis of the combined research suggests sufficient evidence to indicate a link between NAS and cognitive and behavioral difficulties during infancy and through early childhood. Weaknesses in language, deficiencies in cognition, and sometimes attention-deficient hyperactivity disorder could warrant special education services. The research suggests that children exposed to drugs *in utero* are vulnerable to low achievement in school. These children are most often identified as recipients for special education services. It can be concluded from the combination of these studies that early intervention and subsequent intervention are critical in promoting readiness and success in school for children born with NAS. These cognitive and behavioral challenges should be prioritized and addressed in the classroom once these infants reach school age – an added challenge the opioid epidemic is infusing into schools.

Household Addiction and Development

As the research suggests, children born with NAS may have disabilities requiring special education services once they reach school age. Children exposed prenatally to opioids show lower cognitive performance than non-exposed infants and are associated with language weaknesses and cognitive deficiencies (Beckwith & Burke, 2015). Research also indicates that this exposure contributes to the high incidence of neurodevelopmental, cognitive, and behavioral problems (Beckwith & Burke, 2015; Fill et al., 2018; McGlone & Mactier, 2015; Ornoy et al., 2010; Yuan et al., 2014).

In addition to the possibility of cognitive and behavioral challenges for children born with NAS, ample evidence suggests that children living in households experiencing drug abuse may also require additional social, emotional, or academic services in schools. Peisch et al. (2018) reported that children of opioid-addicted individuals have an increased risk of emotional challenges, behavioral problems, and poor social skills, contributing to poor academic performance.

As suggested, the need for academic and behavioral services in schools due to the opioid epidemic is not limited to children born with NAS but also to children born into any family battling addiction. Since living in a household with substance addiction is considered an adverse childhood experience (ACE), children living in opioid-abusing households are at risk for a wide variety of adverse outcomes, including emotional, social, and behavioral disabilities as well as challenges in cognitive and academic functioning (Crouch, 2019). There is an increased risk for negative emotional and behavioral outcomes among children living with a parent with a substance abuse history. The children of parents addicted to opioids are more than twice as likely as their peers to have a drug use problem by young adulthood. Literature suggests that there are developmental problems in children and adolescents living with heroin-addicted mothers even if the children were not born exposed to opioids *in utero* (Gary et al., 2022; Herranz et al., 2014; Nunes et al., 2015).

Additionally, research conducted by Herranz et al. (2014) suggested that children born into opioid-abusing homes may be at risk of developing social problems and psychiatric problems and could have an increased risk of substance abuse in the future. In conclusion, this study determined that children born to heroin-addicted mothers could benefit from close monitoring after birth (Herranz et al., 2014). Nunes et al. (2015) concluded that children born into a family with a substance abuse problem were found to have substantial lifetime issues that would benefit from early intervention, special education services, and outpatient psychological treatment. Both studies suggest that children may need extra support throughout their childhood to minimize the likelihood of social problems, psychological disorders, and substance abuse.

The analysis of the studies indicates that parental opioid addiction has placed many students at risk for academic struggles, which is similar to studies of children born prenatally exposed to opiates. Students exposed to parental drug addiction could also need school-based support services to succeed. Schools must be prepared to address not only the academic needs of these children but also the mental health issues found in children with parents with a history of substance abuse.

In combination of all the literature and available research highlighting the developmental and cognitive impact of household and prenatal opioid exposure on children, a reasonable prediction would be that opioid-crisis regions would have increasing percentages of students who would qualify for special education services once school age. The special education percentages would most likely continue to increase until the overdose numbers start to decrease and the epidemic is under control.

Given the possibility of significant educational implications and the projected increase of children impacted by this public health crisis, what have schools been doing to prepare and address the needs of the students impacted by the opioid epidemic?

Opioid Epidemic and American Schools

The potential implications of the opioid epidemic directly impact children exposed to opioids *in utero* and children in opioid-abusing households. In order to address change with an emphasis on solutions, there needs to be an understanding of what is currently happening in schools, student learning, and the associated educational policies.

The opioid epidemic already has had ramifications in American schools, but the empirical literature on the direct educational impact is limited. Educators feel unprepared and underfunded to address the ramifications of the opioid epidemic (Boulden & Brown, 2022; Lowery et al., 2023). Proactive literature focusing on combating the future of the crisis in the classroom is minimal. Most literature focuses on increased drug education programs nationwide starting at a younger age. There is also literature on the benefits of supplying Narcan in the nurse's office to prevent fatal overdoses in schools.

Policy

Most policy addressing the opioid epidemic comes from the health and community sector, focusing on increasing access to treatment plans, recovery services, and quality intervention centers. However, educational policy leaders have recently added to these efforts by instituting state-level initiatives to support education and prevention efforts. Most states have possession of Narcan in schools and have permission for select medical personnel to administer it (SAMHSA, 2018). In 2019, at least four states (Minnesota, Oregon, South Dakota, and Washington) enacted bills to expand Narcan in schools (Rafa, 2019).

In the United States, almost all 50 states have alcohol and drug abuse education in their middle- and high-school health curriculum. As of 2019, some states, such as Texas, Virginia, Maryland, and Michigan, have opioid misuse as part of the health curriculum.

On September 28, 2018, the U.S. House of Representatives passed the Substance Use-Disorder Prevention that Promotes Opioid Recovery and Treatment for Patients and Communities Act, which includes specific requirements and $50 million in grants per year to support education systems in providing trauma-informed care for students impacted by the opioid crisis. The grant money helps states and school districts increase evidence-based support for students who have experienced trauma (H.R.6, 2018).

Some state-wide initiatives are noteworthy, including programs in Massachusetts, New Hampshire, Ohio, and West Virginia. Here is an overview of a sampling of programs:

Massachusetts: In 2016, a nationally recognized screening program began. The Massachusetts Legislature enacted an Act addressing substance use, treatment, education, and prevention that outlines the requirements for public schools in the Commonwealth to engage in substance use screening and education. Trained staff such as school nurses or counselors began implementing *Screening, Brief Intervention, and Referral to Treatment in Schools (SBIRT)* through the Children's Mental Health Campaign (2021). Often surveyed in middle and high schools, this screening program identified substance abuse in students before it became high risk. Identification is followed by intervention programs or referrals to treatment for students at high risk. The SBIRT mandate became a national model, and numerous agencies are expanding the program and investing in its success (Screening, Brief Intervention, and Referral to Treatment in Schools, 2021).

New Hampshire: In partnership with the New Hampshire Department of Education, the University of New Hampshire Institute on Disability, Antioch University, and the New Hampshire Center for Effective Behavioral Interventions and Support created a multiple-tiered system of supports and behavior wellness (MTSS-B). This multiple-tier model blends behavior interventions with social-emotional learning to address issues such as trauma, student behavior, and mental health – all challenges associated with the opioid crisis in schools. According to the New Hampshire Department of Education website:

> The NH MTSS-B framework ensures that all students are ready to learn. To achieve this, the NH MTSS-B prioritizes universal social-emotional supports through a tiered prevention framework and an integrated mental health delivery system through collaborative family and community partnerships.
>
> (New Hampshire Department of Education, Sect. 3)

Tier 1 is universal support, Tier 2 is targeted supports, and Tier 3 is individualized services. As of 2022, 37 New Hampshire school districts have implemented these supports (New Hampshire Department of Education, 2022).

Ohio: Ohio had several initiatives preventing drug use among youth, including Start Talking! This program invited state troopers, National Guard Members, and law enforcement officers to speak for a few minutes with student leaders. The student leaders were then tasked with presenting the learned information and the benefits of a drug-free lifestyle to peers (Rafa, 2019).

West Virginia: Located in West Virginia, The Martinsburg Initiative used a community-building approach to fight opioid addiction and the cycle of addiction by bringing together and utilizing the police department, school system, higher education, and health care organizations. The goal of the initiative was to break the cycle of addiction and hopefully decrease and mitigate the risk factors for substance abuse, such as adverse childhood experiences (The Martinsburg Initiative, 2020).

Additionally, many of the above state and community initiatives and policies could be supported in schools if President Joe Biden's $20 billion in funding for a new Title 1 Equity Grants program is approved. According to the Department of Education (2022), the proposed grant can potentially incentivize the distribution of school funds with the primary goal of improving equity by distributing resources to support students with high needs. Although the opioid epidemic is not explicitly mentioned, if school districts in opioid-crisis regions qualify, funding could be used to educate the whole child by allocating funds for nonacademic needs, such as prioritizing mental health initiatives and providing funding and support for wraparound services in schools throughout the United States. The grant could also encourage and support trauma-informed practices by providing adequate training to staff. The proposed equity grant would distribute funding to students classified as high needs, such as homeless students, students in foster care, and other disadvantaged students.

Bringing It All Together

Schools find themselves vulnerable to the consequences of the opioid epidemic, contributing to a nationwide educational crisis. Key factors such as the history of opioid distribution, an upsurge in reported opioid abuse within households, and the prevalence of NAS collectively exert influence on educational institutions. Living in a household coping with opioid abuse qualifies as an ACE, presenting an escalating challenge as an increasing number of children arrive at school burdened by additional adverse experiences stemming from household addiction. This situation not only affects the behavioral and cognitive development of these children but also has an influence on the overall school environment. Fully understanding these impacts is in its emerging stages.

The depth of this qualitative study will begin to shed light on the impact through the educator's perspective. Before we dive into the research, Chapter 3 unpacks the ACE study's theoretical framework to understand the foundation of this study.

References

Ahmad, F. B., Cisewski, J. A., Rossen, L. M., & Sutton, P. (2023). *Provisional drug overdose death counts*. National Center for Health Statistics.

Beckwith, A. M., & Burke, S. A. (2015). Identification of early developmental deficits in Infants with prenatal heroin, methadone, and other opioid exposure. *Clinical Pediatrics*, *54*(4), 328.

Boulden, R., & Brown, C. (2022). "We're kind of forgotten": An initial investigation of Appalachian school counselors' lived experiences responding to the opioid crisis. *School Community Journal*, *32*(2), 113–138. https://www.adi.org/journal/2022fw/BouldenBrownFW22.pdf

Carlson, R., Nahhas, R., Martins, S., & Daniulaityte, R. (2016). Predictors of transition to heroin use among initially non-opioid dependent illicit pharmaceutical opioid users: A natural history study. *Drug and Alcohol Dependence*, *160*, 127–134. https://doi.org/10.1016%2Fj.drugalcdep.2015.12.026

Centers for Disease Control and Prevention. (2017). *Number and age-adjusted rates of drug poisoning deaths involving opioid analgesics and heroin: United States, 1999–2014.* https://www.cdc.gov/nchs/data/health_policy/AADR_drug. poisoning_involving_OA_Heroin_US_2000-2014.pdf

Children's Mental Health Campaign. (2021, December 9). *Screening, brief intervention, and referral to treatment for adolescents.* https://www.mass.gov/doc/cmhc-presentation-screening-brief-intervention-and-referral-to-treatment-for-adolescents-12092021-0/download

Crouch, E., Radcliff, E., Hung, P., & Bennett, K. (2019). Challenges to school success and the role of adverse childhood experiences. *Academic Pediatrics*, *19*(8), 899–907. https://doi-org.proxy3.noblenet.org/10.1016/j.acap.2019.08.006

Department of Education. (2022). *Education for the disadvantaged fiscal year 2022 budget request.* https://www2.ed.gov/about/overview/budget/budget22/justifications/a-ed.pdf

Drescher, J., Steyer, L., Townley-Flores, C., & Humphreys, K. (2022). Has the opioid crisis affected student learning? A national analysis of growth rates. *The ANNALS of the American Academy of Political and Social Science*, *703*(1), 234–261. https://doi.org/10.1177/00027162231151524

Drug Enforcement Administration (DEA). (2015). *National drug threat assessment summary.* U.S. Department of Justice.

Felitti, V. J., Anda, R. F., Nordenberg, D., Williamson, D. F., Spitz, A. M., Edwards, V., Koss, M. P., & Marks, J. S. (2019). Relationship of childhood abuse and household dysfunction to many of the leading causes of death in adults: The adverse childhood experiences (ACE) study (reprint). *American Journal of Preventive Medicine*, *56*(6), 774–786. https://doi-org.proxy3.noblenet.org/10.1016/j.amepre.2019.04.001

Fill, M. A., Miller, A. M., Wilkinson, R. H., Warren, M. D., Dunn, J. R., Schaffner, W., & Jones, T. F. (2018). Educational disabilities among children born with neonatal abstinence syndrome. *Pediatrics*, *152*(3), 1–8. https://doi.org/10.1542/peds.2018-0562

Friedman, J., Montero, F., Bourgois, P., Wahbi, R., Dye, D., Goodman-Meza, D., & Shover, C. (2022). Xylazine spreads across the US: A growing component of the increasingly synthetic and polysubstance overdose crisis. *Drug and Alcohol Dependence*, *233*, 109380. https://doi.org/10.1016/j.drugalcdep.2022.109380

Gary, J., Downing, N., & Pittman, A. (2022). The impact of parental opioid use disorder on children in rural Texas. *Substance Use & Misuse*, *57*(8), 1273–1280. https://doi.org/10.1080/10826084.2022.2076879

Haffajee, R. L., & Mello, M. M. (2017). Drug companies' liability for the opioid epidemic. *The New England Journal of Medicine*, *377*(24), 2301–2305. https://doi.org/10.1056/NEJMp1710756

Healthcare Cost and Utilization Project (HCUP). (2021). *HCUP fast stats.* Agency for Healthcare Research and Quality. https://www.hcup-us.ahrq.gov/faststats/NASMap

Hedegaard, H., Chen, L.-H., & Warner, M. (2015). Drug-poisoning deaths involving heroin: United States, 2000–2013. *NCHS Data Brief*, *190*, 1–8.

Hedegaard, H., Miniño, A. M., Spencer, M. R., & Warner, M. (2021, December). *Drug overdose deaths in the United States, 1999–2020.* National Center for Health Statistics.

Herranz, G. S., Vílchez, M. A. L., Ledo, J. D., & Sierra, A. M. (2014). Children born to heroin-addicted mothers: What's the outcome 25 years later? *Journal of Addiction Research and Therapy*, *5*(180).

Hirai, A. H., Ko, J. Y., Owens, P. L., Stocks, C., & Patrick, S. W. (2021). Neonatal abstinence syndrome and maternal opioid-related diagnoses in the US, 2010–2017. *Journal of the American Medical Association*, *325*(2), 146–155. https://doi-org.proxy3.noblenet.org/10.1001/jama.2020.24991

House Amendment to the Senate Amendment, H.R.6, 115th Cong. (2018). https://www.congress.gov/115/bills/hr6/BILLS-115hr6eah.pdf

Humphreys, K., Shover, C. L., Andrews, C. M., Bohnert, A. S. B., Brandeau, M. L., Caulkins, J. P., Chen, J. H., Cuéllar, M.-F., Hurd, Y. L., Juurlink, D. N., Koh, H. K., Krebs, E. E., Lembke, A., Mackey, S. C., Larrimore, L., Suffoletto, B., & Timko, C. (2022). Responding to the opioid crisis in North America and beyond: Recommendations of the Stanford–Lancet Commission. *The Lancet*, *399*(10324), 555–604. https://doi.org/10.1016/s0140-6736(21)02252-2.

Jimenez, M. E., Wade, R., Lin, Y., Morrow, L. M., & Reichman, N. E. (2016). Adverse experiences in early childhood and kindergarten outcomes. *Pediatrics*, *137*(2), 2015–1839.

Jones, C. (2013). Heroin use and heroin use risk behaviors among nonmedical users of prescription opioid pain relievers: United States, 2002–2004 and 2008–2010. *Drug and Alcohol Dependence*, *132*, 95–100.

Kim, H. M., Bone, R. M., McNeill, B., Lee, S. J., Gillon, G., & Woodward, L. J. (2021). Preschool language development of children born to women with an opioid use disorder. *Children*, *8*(4), 268. https://doi.org/10.3390/children8040268.

Lee, S., Bora, S., Austin, N., Westerman, A., & Henderson, J. (2020). Neurodevelopmental outcomes of children born to opioid-dependent mothers: A systematic review and meta-analysis. *Academic Pediatrics*, *20*(3), 308–318. https://doi.org/10.1016/j.acap.2019.11.005

Lowery, C. L., Hess, M. E., Ramsey, C. K. G., & Fewell, C. (2023). Opioids and school leaders: Bricolage leadership in Appalachian Ohio. *International Journal of Leadership in Education*. https://doi.org/10.1080/13603124.2023.2275642

The Martinsburg Initiative. (2020). https://themartinsburginitiative.com/

McGlone, L., & Mactier, H. (2015). Infants of opioid-dependent mothers: Neurodevelopment at six months. *Early Human Development*, *91*(1), 19–21.

Muhuri, P., Gfroerer, J., & Davies, M., (2013). *Associations of Nonmedical Pain Reliever Use and Initiation of Heroin Use in the United States*. CBHSQ Data Review, Substance Abuse and Mental Health Services Administration (SAMHSA). https://www.samhsa.gov/data/sites/default/files/DR006/DR006/nonmedical-pain-reliever-use-2013.htm

National Center for Health Statistics. (2021, November 17). *Drug overdose deaths in the U.S. top 100,000 annually*. Center of Disease Control and Prevention. https://www.cdc.gov/nchs/pressroom/nchs_press_releases/2021/20211117.htm

National Conference of State Legislatures (NCSL). (2019). *Prescribing policies: States confront opioid overdose epidemic*. https://www.ncsl.org/research/health/prescribing-policies-states-confront-opioid-overdose-epidemic.aspx

National Institute on Drug Abuse (NIDA). (2021, June 1). *Fentanyl drugfacts*. https://nida.nih.gov/research-topics/trends-statistics/overdose-death-rates

New Hampshire Department of Education. (2022). *NH's multi-tiered system of support for behavioral health and wellness model (MTSS-B)*. www.education.nh.gov

Nunes, E., Weissman, M., Goldsten, R., McAvay, G., Beckford, C., Seracini, A., & Wickramaratne, P. (2015). Psychiatric disorders and impairment in the children of opiate addicts: Prevalence and distribution by ethnicity. *American Journal on Addictions*, *9*(3), 232–241.

Nygaard, E., Moe, V., Slinning, K., & Walhoyd, K. (2015). Longitudinal cognitive development of children born to mothers with opioid and polysubstance use. *Pediatric Research*, *78*(3), 330–335.

O'Donnell, M., Nassar, N., Leonard, H., Hagan, R., Mathews, R., Patterson, Y., & Stanley, F. (2009). The increasing prevalence of neonatal withdrawal syndrome is a population study of maternal factors and child protection involvement. *Pediatrics*, *123*(4), e614–e621. https://doi.org/10.1542/peds.2008-2888

Ornoy, A., Daka, L., Goldzweig, G., Gil, Y., Mjen, L., Levit, S., Shufman, E., Bar-Hamburger, R., & Greenbaum, C. (2010). Neurodevelopmental and psychological assessment of adolescents born to drug-addicted parents: Effects of SES and adoption. *Child Abuse & Neglect*, *34*(5), 354–368.

Patrick, S. W., Davis, M. M., Lehman, C. U., & Cooper, W. O. (2015). Increasing incidence and geographic distribution of neonatal abstinence syndrome: The United States 2009 to 2012. *Journal of Perinatology*, *35*(8), 667. https://doi.org/10.1038/jp.2015.63

Paulozzi, L. J., Mack, K. A., Hockenberry, J. M., & Division of Unintentional Injury Prevention, National Center for Injury Prevention and Control, CDC. (2014). Vital signs: Variation among states prescribing opioid pain relievers and benzodiazepines–United States, 2012. *Morbidity and Mortality Weekly Report*, *63*(26), 563–568.

Peisch, V., Sullivan, A. D., Breslend, N. L., Benoit, R., Sigmon, S. C., Forehand, G. L., Strolin-Goltzman, J., & Forehand, R. (2018). Parental opioid abuse: A review of child outcomes, parenting, and parenting interventions. *Journal of Child and Family Studies*, *27*(7), 2082–2099. https://doi.org/10.1007/s10826-018-1061-0

Pollini, R. A., Banta-Green, C. J., Cuevas-Mota, J., Metzner, M., Teshale, E., & Garfein, R.S. (2011). Problematic use of prescription-type opioids prior to heroin use among heroin injectors. *Substance Abuse and Rehabilitation*, *2*(1), 173–180.

Rafa, A. (2019). *Policy analysis: The status of school discipline in state policy*. Education Commission of the States.

Scholl, S., Rudd, R., & Bacon, S. (2018). Overdose deaths involving opioids, cocaine, and psychostimulants – United States, 2015–2016. *MMWR Morb Mortal Wkly Rep*, *67*, 349–358. http://dx.doi.org/10.15585/mmwr.mm6712a1external icon.

Screening, Brief Intervention, and Referral to Treatment in Schools. (2021). *Massachusetts screening, brief, intervention, and referral to treatment training & technical assistance*. https://masbirt.org/schools/

Seth, P., Scholl, L., Rudd, R. A., & Bacon, S. (2018). Overdose Deaths Involving Opioids, Cocaine, and Psychostimulants – United States, 2015–2016. *MMWR. Morbidity and mortality weekly report*, *67*(12), 349–358. https://doi.org/10.15585/mmwr.mm6712a1

Substance Abuse and Mental Health Services. (2018). *Opioid overdose prevention toolkit (HHS Publication No. SMA18-1472)*. U.S. Department of Health and Human Resources. https://store.samhsa.gov/system/files/sma18-4742.pdf

Trump, D. (2017, October 2). *Remarks by President Trump on combatting drug demand and the opioid crisis*. White House Archives. https://trumpwhitehouse.archives.gov/briefings-statements/remarks-president-trump-combatting-drug-demand-opioid-crisis/

United States Press Release. (2017, October 27). *HHS acting secretary declares public health emergency to address national opioid crisis*. https://public3.pagefreezer.com/content/HHS.gov/31-12-2020T08:51/https://www.hhs.gov/about/news/2017/10/26/hhs-acting-secretary-declares-public-health-emergency-address-national-opioid-crisis.html

Winkelman, T., Villapiano, N., Kozhimannil, K. B., Davis, M. M., & Patrick, S. W. (2018). Incidence and costs of neonatal abstinence syndrome among infants with Medicaid: 2004–2014. *Pediatrics*, *141*(4), e20173520. https://doi.org/10.1542/peds.2017-3520

Wolf, P., Ponicki, W., Kepple, N. J., & Gaidus, A. (2016, September). Are community-level prescription opioid overdoses associated with child harm? A spatial analysis of California zip codes, 2001–2011. *Drug and Alcohol Dependence*, *166*, 202–208. https://doi.org/10.1016/j.drugalcdep.2016.07.014.

WONDER. (2021). *Wide-ranging online data for epidemiologic research Atlanta, GA: CDC*. Centers for Disease Control and Prevention. http://wonder.cdc.gov

WONDER. (2023). *Wide-ranging online data for epidemiologic research Atlanta, GA: CDC*. Centers for Disease Control and Prevention. http://wonder.cdc.gov

Yuan, Q., Rubic, M., Seah, J., Rae, C., Wright, I. M., Kaltenbach, K., Feller, J. M., Abdel-Latif, M. E., Chu, C., & Oei, J. L. (2014). Do maternal opioids reduce neonatal regional brain volumes? A pilot study. *Journal of Perinatology*, *34*(12), 909–913. https://doi.org/10.1038/jp.2014.111

3 Beyond the Crisis

Unraveling the Impact of Adverse Childhood Experiences and Opioid Exposure on Education

> The impact of the opioid epidemic is intense and is seen here through extreme behaviors. Kids are clearly living with trauma. Many kindergartners this year have come in from situations where you can see the direct effect of a mother or father who's incarcerated, mother and father who are addicts, kindergartners who have come in under the care of other relatives that have communicated to us that addiction is part of the issue. Or already part of the foster care program, or under state custody. And we've seen a real increase this year in not just troublesome, problematic behaviors, but very extreme behaviors from children who are clearly in crisis from the trauma of dealing with this epidemic in their everyday lives.
>
> – Nelson, Massachusetts Assistant Principal

The intricate interplay between adverse childhood experiences (ACEs) and children's environmental and household exposure to opioid addiction and opioid-use disorder can significantly impact the cognitive, emotional, and academic trajectory of children. Understanding the convergence of these phenomena aims to illuminate the ramifications within the schools.

ACEs are potentially traumatic events that can negatively impact a person's health and well-being throughout their lifetime. This includes maltreatment, neglect, abuse, and living in an environment that harms one's development, such as household substance abuse, divorce, criminal behavior, and incarceration. Children residing in opioid-using environments, communities, and households are more at risk of exposure to adversity and may experience multiple ACEs. Such experiences and exposures may impact and influence the child's educational trajectory and the additional resources a school system needs to provide for academic development and success for students with ACEs. The ACE study is the theoretical framework of the study.

DOI: 10.4324/9781003378204-4

Adverse Childhood Experiences and Household and Community Opioid Exposure

The role that stress has on a child's brain development and cognitive and social growth is often cited as a critical factor in why children living with adverse life experiences perform poorly in school. The stress of such adverse childhood experiences has been known to disrupt the developing brain. Stress alters a child's language, social, and cognitive development and is not easily controlled by educators because so much of it derives from family life and events outside of school (Jensen, 2009). Understanding how children experience the opioid epidemic is critical to understanding the influence it has on students' behaviors at school.

ACEs were first described in medical health outcomes in a study by CDC-Kaiser in 1998. Since that study was published, other studies have looked into ACEs' impact on mental health, behavior, life opportunities, resilience, and economic stability. Adverse childhood experiences include emotional, physical, and sexual abuse. Household challenges such as the mother being treated violently, household substance abuse, mental illness, parental separation or divorce, and households involved in criminal behavior are considered adverse childhood experiences. Additionally, emotional and physical neglect are also ACEs.

ACEs are extremely common, and the original CDC-Kaiser ACE study found that 64% of participants had at least one ACE.

Understanding what defines an ACE is functional in understanding the implications. There are proven short-term and long-term adverse consequences for a person's health and well-being. There is growing evidence that supports the initial CDC study and indicates that toxic stress, such as repeated adverse experiences, can cause permanent damage to the developing brain and alter the functioning of the immune, neurological, and endocrine systems in individuals, which could predispose them to high risks of disease and even early death. Unfortunately, there appears to be an evolving cycle of exposure to parental opioid abuse during childhood that has been linked to increased risk for adolescent substance abuse and suicide (Biederman et al., 2000; Brent et al., 2019; Gibbons et al., 2021; Griesler et al., 2019). These studies support the suggestion that the ongoing opioid crisis in this country has far-reaching and adverse societal effects, particularly on children, as they are exposed to associated ACEs related to the opioid epidemic.

The ACE Pyramid

The ACE Pyramid was derived from the CDC-Kaiser Permanente Adverse Childhood Experiences Study (2014) and explains the "mechanism by which adverse childhood experiences influence health and well-being throughout the lifespan" (CDC, 2014).

The pyramid illustrates adverse childhood experiences that can lead to disrupted neurodevelopment and social, emotional, and cognitive impairments. The disruption in neurodevelopment may result in social, emotional, cognitive, and health impairments that directly influence the child's educational experiences and increase the need for academic, social, emotional, and behavioral interventions once in school. Additionally, as students get older, such life experiences add to the likelihood of health risk behaviors and disease, disability, and social problems. It was found that these adverse experiences increase the chance of an early death.

According to the CDC-Kaiser Permanente Adverse Childhood Experiences Study (2014), a household member who misuses drugs qualifies as an adverse childhood experience. Additionally, the literature suggests that children who experience trauma, neglect, abuse, and abandonment all have increased chances of emotional, behavioral, and cognitive disabilities and would require educational interventions (Herranz et al., 2014; Nunes et al., 2015).

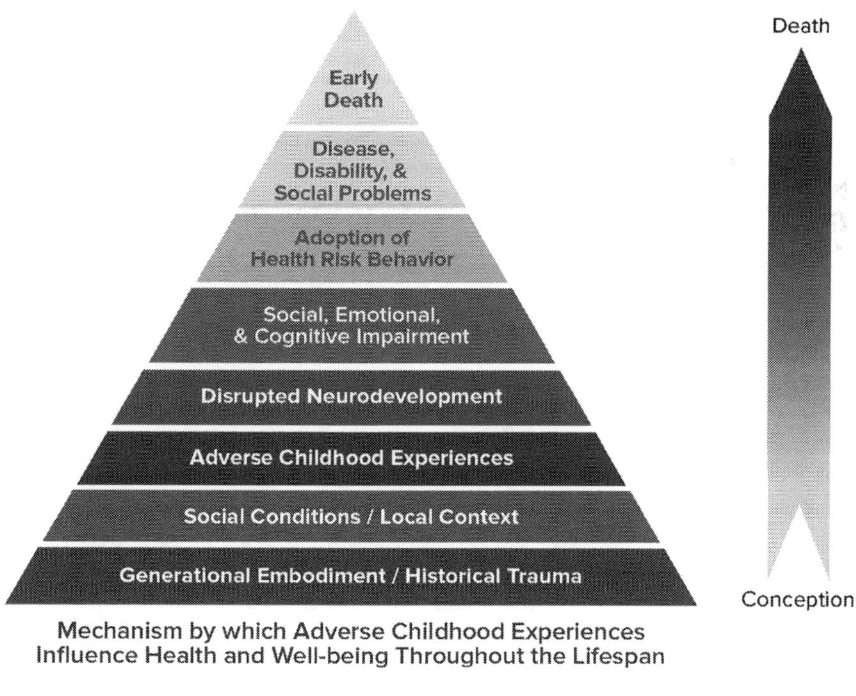

Figure 3.1 The ACE Pyramid model

Source: https://www.cdc.gov/violenceprevention/aces/about.html

ACE's and School Struggles

Literature reveals that parental opioid addiction has placed many students at risk for school failure and academic struggles. Students exposed to parental drug addiction could require school-based support services to succeed in school (Crouch, 2019; Darolia et al., 2020; Drescher et al., 2022; Herranz et al., 2014; Jimenez et al., 2016; Nunes et al., 2015; Peisch et al., 2018).

There is ample evidence that children with ACE have a greater incidence of challenges in school (Crouch, 2019). ACEs can affect student learning and behavior in the classroom (Zhang & Mersky, 2022). According to the CDC-Kaiser Permanente Adverse Childhood Experiences Study, children with three or more ACEs are five times more likely to have attendance issues, six times more likely to have behavior problems, and three times more likely to experience academic failure (Felitti et al., 2019 & Kaiser Permanente Thriving Schools, n.d.). Furthermore, according to Harvard University's Center for the Developing Child (2022), when a person experiences frequent, intense, or prolonged adversity, such as caregiver's substance abuse, exposure to violence, chronic neglect, or physical or emotional abuse, it can result in profound adverse effects on the mind and body that can impact health and learning. The stress of such adverse childhood experiences has been known to disrupt the developing brain, leading to toxic amounts of stress.

Children exposed to higher levels of neighborhood violence have worse education outcomes than children who are less exposed (Sharkey et al., 2012), concluding that childhood exposure to the consequences of the opioid epidemic may result in negative education outcomes (Harding et al., 2010; Sharkey, 2013).

Childhood environmental conditions such as ACEs and exposure are also linked to the formation of a child's executive functioning abilities (defined as mental capacities associated with working memory, inhibitory control, and cognitive or mental flexibility) and are considered not only critical in early childhood but also necessary for healthy development through adolescence (Center for the Developing Child, 2022). Additionally, research has shown that chaotic and stressful environments, such as living in a home with substance abuse, can inhibit executive functioning development and that environments lacking healthy parent–child relationships can dampen the development of executive capacities (Barkley, 2001; Evans & Wachs, 2010). Therefore, traumatic or prolonged exposure to stress, such as substance abuse, can lead to toxic stress and can change the architecture of a child's developing brain, changes that can have lasting effects on physiological, cognitive, behavioral, and psychological functioning (Juster et al., 2010; McEwen & Gianaros, 2010).

Evidence from various studies supports the original CDC-Kaiser results from 1998. Household exposure can also impact critical education tasks such as executive functioning abilities. Executive functioning tasks include working memory, cognitive flexibility, organization, attention span, and impulse control. Research has shown that stressful environments can impact the development of executive functioning (Barkley, 2001; Lengua et al., 2007).

In addition to exposure to addiction in the household, children are exposed to the ramifications of opioid addiction in their communities. Evidence and literature show that negative home and community factors can be associated with a loss of learning opportunities. Children exposed to high levels of toxic stress and community violence in their neighborhoods have worse educational outcomes than those not exposed (Sharkey et al., 2013; Shonkoff & Garner, 2012). The literature and research suggest that childhood exposure to toxic stress and neighborhood violence associated with the opioid epidemic, whether that exposure is in the home, neighborhood, community, or school, may result in negative education outcomes.

Children living in opioid-abusing households and communities are more at risk of exposure to such adversity and may experience multiple adverse childhood experiences. Such experiences and exposures could impact and influence the child's educational trajectory along with the resources a school system needs to provide for academic progression and success. The ACE study is the theoretical framework of this study. It is used as a roadmap for understanding the overall impact of the opioid crisis on students and schools in regions and communities in crisis.

Bringing It All Together

ACEs are potentially traumatic events that can negatively impact a person's health and well-being throughout their lifetime. This includes situations children may experience when exposed to the ramifications of the opioid epidemic, such as maltreatment, neglect, and abuse. Living in an environment that is harmful to one's development, such as household substance abuse, divorce, household criminal behavior, and incarceration, also happens when children are exposed to an epicenter of the opioid crisis. Children in opioid-abusing households are more at risk of exposure to such adversity and may experience multiple ACEs. Such experiences and exposures could impact and influence the child's educational trajectory along with the resources a school system needs to provide for academic progression and success. As the research is shared, analyzed, and discussed, the ACE study magnifies how adverse childhood experiences influence the developing child and how ACEs impact children's learning and school experience. There is sufficient evidence that children from disadvantaged backgrounds, such as living in a community and home challenged by addiction, could experience lost learning opportunities and increased social, emotional, and cognitive challenges that other children may not experience.

References

Barkley, R. A. (2001). The executive functions and self-regulation: An evolutionary neuropsychological perspective. *Neuropsychology Review*, *11*(1), 1–29. https://doi.org/10.1023/A:1009085417776

Biederman, J., Faraone, S. V., Monuteaux, M. C., & Feighner, J. A. (2000). Patterns of alcohol and drug use in adolescents can be predicted by parental substance use disorders. *Pediatrics*, *106*(4), 792–797. https://doi.org/10.1542/peds.106.4.792

Brent, D. A., Hur, K., & Gibbons, R. D. (2019). Association between parental medical claims for opioid prescriptions and risk of suicide attempt by their children. *Journal of the American Medical Association*, *Psychiatry*, *76*(9), 1–7.

Center for the Developing Child. (2022). *Toxic stress*. Harvard University. https://developingchild.harvard.edu/science/key-concepts/toxic-stress/

Centers for Disease Control and Prevention. (2014). *The ACE pyramid*. National Center for Injury Prevention and Control, Division of Violence Prevention. https://www.cdc.gov/violenceprevention/acestudy/about.html

Crouch, E., Radcliff, E., Hung, P., & Bennett, K. (2019). Challenges to school success and the role of adverse childhood experiences. *Academic Pediatrics*, *19*(8), 899–907. https://doi-org.proxy3.noblenet.org/10.1016/j.acap.2019.08.006

Darolia, R., Owens, S., & Tyler, J. (2020). *The opioid crisis and educational performance* (Working Paper No. 20-322). Annenberg Institute at Brown University. https://doi.org/10.26300/s2j8-r106

Drescher, J., Steyer, L., Townley-Flores, C., & Humphreys, K. (2022). Has the opioid crisis affected student learning? A national analysis of growth rates. *The ANNALS of the American Academy of Political and Social Science*, *703*(1), 234–261. https://doi.org/10.1177/00027162231151524

Evans, G. W., & Wachs, T. D. (Eds.). (2010). *Chaos and its influence on children's development: An ecological perspective*. American Psychological Association. https://doi.org/10.1037/12057-000

Felitti, V. J., Anda, R. F., Nordenberg, D., Williamson, D. F., Spitz, A. M., Edwards, V., Koss, M. P., & Marks, J. S. (2019). Relationship of childhood abuse and household dysfunction to many of the leading causes of death in adults: The adverse childhood experiences (ACE) study (reprint). *American Journal of Preventive Medicine*, *56*(6), 774–786. https://doi-org.proxy3.noblenet.org/10.1016/j.amepre.2019.04.001

Gibbons, R. D., Hur, K., & Quinn, P. D. (2021). Concomitant opioid and benzodiazepine use and risk of suicide attempt and intentional self-harm: Pharmacoepidemiologic study. *Drug and Alcohol Dependence*, *228*, 109046. https://doi.org/10.1016/j.drugalcdep.2021.109046

Griesler, P. C., Hu, M. C., Wall, M. M., & Kandel, D. B. (2019). Nonmedical prescription opioid use by parents and adolescents in the US. *Pediatrics*, *143*(3), e20182354. https://doi.org/10.1542/peds.2018-2354

Harding, D. J., Gennetian, L., Winship, C., Sanbonmatsu, L., & Kling, J. R. (2010). *Unpacking neighborhood influences on education outcomes: Setting the stage for future research* (NBER Working Paper No. 16055). National Bureau of Economic Research. http://www.nber.org/papers/w16055

Herranz, G. S., Vílchez, M. A. L., Ledo, J. D., & Sierra, A. M. (2014). Children born to heroin-addicted mothers: What's the outcome 25 years later? *Journal of Addiction Research and Therapy*, *5*(180). https://doi.org/10.4172/2155-6105.1000180

Jensen, E. (2009). *Teaching with poverty in mind: What being poor does to kids' minds and what schools can do about it.* Association for Supervision and Curriculum Development.

Jimenez, M. E., Wade, R., Jr., Lin, Y., Morrow, L. M., & Reichman, N. E. (2016). Adverse experiences in early childhood and kindergarten outcomes. *Pediatrics*, *137*(2), e20151839.

Juster, R. P., McEwen, B. S., & Lupien, S. J. (2010). Allostatic load biomarkers of chronic stress and impact on health and cognition. *Neuroscience and Biobehavioral Reviews*, *35*(1), 2–16. https://doi.org/10.1016/j.neubiorev.2009.10.002

Kaiser Permanente Thriving Schools (n.d). Adverse Childhood Expereriences retrieved from: https://thrivingschools.kaiserpermanente.org/mental-health/aces/

Lengua, L. J., Honorado, E., & Bush, N. R. (2007). Contextual risk and parenting as predictors of effortful control and social competence in preschool children. *Journal of Applied Developmental Psychology*, *28*(1), 40–55. https://doi.org/10.1016/j.appdev.2006.10.001

McEwen, B. S., & Gianaros, P. J. (2010). Central role of the brain in stress and adaptation: Links to socioeconomic status, health, and disease. *Annals of the New York Academy of Sciences*, *1186*, 190–222. https://doi.org/10.1111/j.1749-6632.2009.05331.x

Nunes, E., Weissman, M., Goldsten, R., McAvay, G., Beckford, C., Seracini, A., & Wickramaratne, P. (2015). Psychiatric disorders and impairment in the children of opiate addicts: Prevalence and distribution by ethnicity. *American Journal on Addictions*, *9*(3), 232–241.

Peisch, V., Sullivan, A. D., Breslend, N. L., Benoit, R., Sigmon, S. C., Forehand, G. L., Strolin-Goltzman, J., & Forehand, R. (2018). Parental opioid abuse: A review of child outcomes, parenting, and parenting interventions. *Journal of Child and Family Studies*, *27*(7), 2082–2099. https://doi.org/10.1007/s10826-018-1061-0

Sharkey, P. T., Schwartz, A. E., Ellen, I. G., & Lacoe, J. (2013). *High stakes in the classroom, high stakes on the street: The effects of community violence on students' standardized test performance* (Working Paper No. 03-13). IESP, NYU Steinhardt School of Culture, Education, and Human Development.

Sharkey, P. T., Tirado-Strayer, N., Papachristos, A. V., & Raver, C. C. (2012). The effect of local violence on children's attention and impulse control. *American Journal of Public Health*, *102*(12), 2287–2293.

Shonkoff, J., & Garner, A. (2012). The lifelong effects of early childhood adversity and toxic stress. *Pediatrics*, *129*(1), e232–e246. https://doi.org/10.1542/peds.2011-2663

Zhang, L., & Mersky, J. P. (2022). Bidirectional relations between adverse childhood experiences and children's behavioral problems. *Child & Adolescent Social Work Journal*, *39*(2), 183–193. https://doi.org/10.1007/s10560-020-00720-1

4 Research Methodology

A Comprehensive Multiple-Case-Study Exploration of Elementary Schools in Opioid-Crisis Regions of the Northeastern United States

> I think that during the day you put on a happy face, because you know it's what the kids need to see, but then it affects you at home. Ya know, coming here and hearing about sexual abuse, and how the children have no food, and how they get food and hide it underneath . . . it's just . . . it is so wearing on everyone here, emotionally. You do become numb to it, bed bugs and lice are a daily occurrence. It's just kind of, you know, do I send a kid that has lice to the nurse every day? Because they get sent home and I don't want them sent home, or do I keep them where they need to be fed, warm, safe? So, it's a constant struggle emotionally, not to . . . you know, you wanna save them. I've brought in clothes, I've brought in food, I've had my kids go through their toys. I fed one girl for four months at lunch last year, given my own lunch to kids, just to have them make it through the day and feel something. It's wearing. I think the trauma that . . . especially this school, the teachers and administrators feel is like nothing that I've ever seen before and you know it's because of this horrible epidemic.
>
> –Andrea, New Hampshire K-2 Special Education Teacher

The adverse childhood experience (ACE) study progressively uncovered how ACEs are strongly connected to the development and prevalence of risk factors for disease, health, and social well-being throughout a person's lifespan (Centers for Disease Control and Prevention, 2012).

The impact that ACEs have on a child's well-being, from historical trauma, social conditions, adverse life experiences leading to disrupted neurodevelopment, and social, emotional, and cognitive impairments, is critically important in this study because outside traumas can adversely impact a child's mental and social learning and educational experience in the school setting. The community and household experiences of students can affect the educators who work with them daily.

The ACE Pyramid's framework served as a roadmap for this study to explain and predict the impact the opioid epidemic may have on schools in crisis regions where trauma's impact the developing child. For example, household substance-use disorder, parent incarceration, abuse, and neglect

DOI: 10.4324/9781003378204-5

could all be ramifications and experiences a child exposed to opioid addiction could suffer.

A hypothesis of this study based on the ACE study is that the experiences of children in the community and household are brought to schools in opioid-crisis regions and impact the functions of learning and the operation of the school. Another theory is that there could be an increase in students who qualify for special education because social, cognitive, and emotional impairments in children increase when experiencing frequent traumas.

Before findings are revealed and discussed as they apply to the ACE study and beyond, the research method, design, procedure, sampling, and data analysis of the study are shared.

Multiple-Case Study

The multiple-case-study design offers a proven tool for achieving a deep understanding of the specific phenomenon – the impact of the opioid epidemic on schools located in opioid-crisis regions of the United States. Using the multiple-case-study design will be beneficial to identify themes and patterns among selected schools in crisis regions. It may provide a general understanding of the ramifications of the opioid epidemic on elementary schools regardless of the state. Commonly occurring similarities, frequencies, and patterns will be identified in the various locations.

The research design for this study was a multiple-case-study design. Yin (2018) defined a case study as "an empirical method that investigates a contemporary phenomenon in depth and within the real-world context" (p.15), while Stake (1995) defined a case study as "the study of the particularity and complexity of a single case, coming to understand its activity within important circumstances" (p. xi). This particular case study investigated the phenomenon and its unique complexities while documenting the details of its contexts. The multiple-case-study design will rely on various sources of evidence, with different collected data to "converge in triangulating fashion" (Yin, 2018, p. 15). Additionally, the multiple-case-study research design served as a tool for a deep understanding of this phenomenon by uncovering consistent patterns and themes that schools within opioid-crisis regions are experiencing. The study aims to understand a real-world situation experienced by schools as a direct result of the opioid epidemic.

Research Questions

In this study, the consequences of the opioid epidemic, teacher preparedness, experiences, and impact on education will be highlighted and analyzed. The research questions measured awareness and the effects of the ramifications of the opioid epidemic. The research questions for this study are as follows:

1. How is the opioid epidemic impacting elementary schools in opioid-crisis regions of the Northeast?
2. How are schools located in opioid-crisis regions proactively preparing for the influx of students affected by the opioid epidemic entering the school?
3. How are schools in opioid-crisis regions developing and implementing professional development for administrators, teachers, and school staff to address the needs of students impacted by the opioid crisis?

The research purposefully raised consciousness about the importance of awareness and planning, the experiences of educators working in crisis regions in the United States, the significance of professional development and training, and increased teachers' consciousness and knowledge of student needs in opioid-crisis regions.

The study included multiple forms of evidence collected, including interviews and questionnaires from various professionals in different roles working in schools in opioid-crisis regions. Teachers might view their experiences, knowledge, and preparedness differently from other teachers in the same or different school districts. Teachers' words were documented throughout the interviews, and open-ended survey collection and perspectives were recorded. As Creswell (2013) explained:

> Qualitative researchers conduct a study intending to report multiple realities when studying individuals. Evidence of multiple realities includes using multiple forms of evidence in themes using the actual words of different individuals and presenting different perspectives.
>
> (Creswell, 2013, p. 20)

Given the nature of this study, the methodology employed, and the research goal (to explain the phenomenon rather than predict the outcome), philosophical assumptions were identified to maximize the strengths of the study design and the multiple realities of participants. The embedded ontological issue relates to the nature of the participant's existence and its characteristics. At the same time, epistemological assumptions embrace minimizing the distance between the researcher and those being researched. Accordingly, the research relied on quotes as evidence, and the study took place on location. Interviews were conducted in the "field" where the participants work, in schools located in opioid-crisis regions.

Experiencing the atmosphere of the participants and the environmental influences may intensify the knowledge and understanding of the phenomenon. Listening and engaging in the worlds of participants while observing the emotions and ecological consequences that impact the circumstances surrounding the phenomenon may affect objectivity. Exposure to the opioid-impacted environment will influence the detachment of the situation but also create essential contexts for understanding what the participants are saying and referring to during interviews.

Participants and Sampling

The participants for this research study were located in public schools in the Northeastern United States. Each of the public schools is located in an identified opioid-crisis region. Specifically, three school districts in three different Northeast states were investigated. The chosen districts within each state are located in areas where overdose rates are considerably above the national average.

Massachusetts, New Hampshire, and Maine have been identified as having sizeable geographical opioid-crisis regions within the state. Therefore, the three school districts investigated are located in Massachusetts, New Hampshire, and Maine. Districts were chosen within each state because the cities/towns in the districts were in opioid crisis areas. Specifically, crisis areas are identified through data released by the Centers for Disease Control.

Each investigated region qualified for participation in the case study through identification as having significantly higher overdose rates per 100,000 people than the national average. The Centers for Disease Control and Prevention (2015) considered more than 30 overdose deaths per 100,000 people within a year as a foundational criterion for a high-crisis area beyond the national average. Within each region, a city or town was identified as a significant contributor to the high overdose rates. Overdose data was analyzed based on information available at the Centers for Disease Control. Specifically, the school district within the identified city was the district involved in the research. This criterion was applied to three districts that qualified for this study. Once districts were identified and access was granted, a school was identified within each city/town as the focus of the case study. The particular school was identified through district administrator recommendations and access approval.

Surveys were distributed to every staff member who qualified. The participants in each school were school administrators, special education chairpersons/administrators/teachers, social workers, counselors, consultants, and kindergarten through second-grade teachers. The survey investigates the impact of the opioid epidemic in the classroom. It explores teachers, counselors, and administrators' comfort level in educating students exposed to traumatizing situations and social, emotional, and cognitive disabilities due to the ramifications of their exposure to the opioid crisis. Additionally, interviews took place within the schools based on survey results and participants willing to be interviewed. Interview questions were strategically developed and took an in-depth look at experiences and comforts based on an analysis of survey data. Other personnel, such as administrators, special education directors, and counselors, were interviewed to develop a holistic understanding of the impact the opioid epidemic was having on the school, teachers, and leadership of the school. In addition to interviews and surveys, various data such as documents, district professional development plans, and archival information were obtained from other sources to triangulate and combine all information to draw conclusions and generate themes.

Research Design, Procedure, and Data Analysis

The case-study design, procedure, and data analysis follow Yin's (2018) multiple-case-study method, specifically using replication logic. Replication logic is "the logic for selecting two or more cases in a multiple-case study" (Yin, 2018, p. 288). Selecting two or more cases is to confirm or deny predictions that cases may have different or similar findings. When using replication logic, if all or most cases provide similar results, there can be substantial support for developing a preliminary theory that describes a phenomenon (Eisenhardt, 1989). Figure 4.1 demonstrates the research procedure by defining the theory and design leading to the initial preparation of the three cases. The illustration shows the data collection, analysis, and individual case report as the next steps in the research design. Subsequently, the concluding cross-case analysis, development of policy implications, and conclusion are established within the illustration.

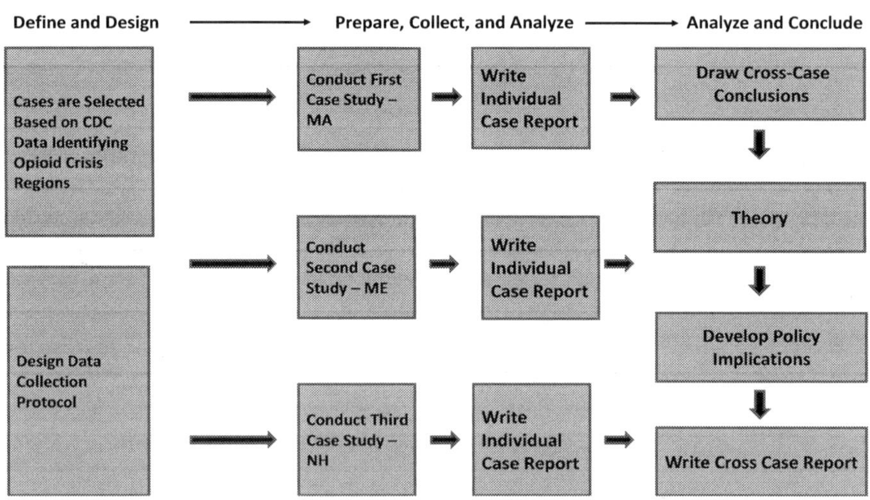

Figure 4.1 Research procedure

Data Collection Protocol

According to Stake (1995), "There is no particular moment when data collection begins. It begins before there is a commitment to make the study: backgrounding, acquaintance with other cases, first impressions" (p. 49). In these cases, data collection began once the sites were determined and access granted. Each of the three case-study sites in each state had the same protocol. The data collection protocol occurred as follows:

Step 1: The first step was an initial discussion with a district administrator to gain access to the school district and school. This was an informal discussion to explain the purpose of the research, gain approval, discuss the plan, and ask to be directed to a recommended school within the district for the case study. The study also was submitted to district-wide Internal Review Boards (IRBs) for approval. At this time, access to documents such as professional development minutes and professional development agendas for the current academic year and previous years was requested. The request was specific to district-wide documents and specific school-based documents, if available. Archival records were also accessed, such as special education data. The archival data was public information and could be accessed through the various Department of Education websites.

Step 2: Once access to a school was gained, a questionnaire was sent to all kindergarten through second-grade teachers and other professionals who work with students. The questionnaire asked explicitly about the professional's history, experiences, professional development opportunities, experiences negotiating the opioid epidemic, and other demographic information. It used a Likert scale and open-ended questions. The questionnaire also established interviews based on willingness to participate and the survey responses.

Step 3: Based on questionnaire results, interviews with teachers were conducted. The first interviews were of kindergarten through second-grade teachers in each case study. Interviews were to include at least five teachers per school district until a complete saturation of understanding was collected. Within the semi-structured interview, access was requested to any other pertinent documents at the school.

All interviews were audio recorded and transcribed verbatim.

The following are the educators' interview questions:

1. How has the opioid epidemic affected your classroom/school?
2. What is your school/district doing to proactively prepare you for the influx of students that will be entering your classroom/school that will have been exposed to the opioid epidemic (born addicted to opioids/living in a home devastated by opioids)?

3. What is your school doing to develop and implement professional development to address the needs of students impacted by the opioid epidemic?
4. How familiar are you with the special education needs, such as social-emotional, behavioral, and cognitive disabilities of children affected by the opioid epidemic? Explain
5. Have special education services and referrals been affected or changed due to the opioid epidemic? Explain.
6. How is your school supporting the needs of students affected by the opioid crisis? Explain.
7. If you have any stories to share about the effects of the opioid epidemic on your classroom/school/or district, please share.

Step 4: Once the teacher/educator/counselor interviews were complete, the special education administrator and a school administrator, such as the principal or the vice principal, were interviewed. Within the semi-structured interview, access was requested to any other pertinent documents that the school was willing to share. These were also the interview questions for support staff such as counselors, social workers, and mental health providers.

The following are the school administrators' interview questions:

1. How has the opioid epidemic affected your school? District?
2. What is your school/district doing to proactively prepare administrators and teachers for the influx of students that will have been exposed to the opioid epidemic (born addicted to opioids/living in a home devastated by opioids)?
3. What is your school doing to develop and implement professional development to address the needs of students impacted by the opioid epidemic?
4. How familiar are you with the special education needs, such as social-emotional, behavioral, and cognitive disabilities of children affected by the opioid epidemic? Explain
5. Have special education services and referrals been affected or changed due to the opioid epidemic? Explain.
6. How is your school supporting the needs of students affected by the opioid crisis? Explain.
7. If you have any stories to share about the effects of the opioid epidemic on your school or district, please share.

Step 5: The final interview with the district administrator from the initial informal meeting in Step 1 was requested. Within the semi-structured interview, access to any other pertinent documents that the school was willing to share was requested.

The following are the district administrators' interview questions:

1. How has the opioid epidemic affected your school? District?
2. What is your school/district doing to proactively prepare administrators and teachers for the influx of students that will have been exposed to the opioid epidemic (born addicted to opioids/living in a home devastated by opioids)?
3. What is your school doing to develop and implement professional development to address the needs of students impacted by the opioid epidemic?
4. How familiar are you with the special education needs, such as social-emotional, behavioral, and cognitive disabilities of children affected by the opioid epidemic? Explain
5. Have special education services and referrals been affected or changed due to the opioid epidemic? Explain.
6. How is your school supporting the needs of students affected by the opioid crisis? Explain.
7. If you have any stories to share about the effects of the opioid epidemic on your school or district, please share.

Step 6: Analysis the results (detailed explanation below) and repeat these steps at each participating case-study site.

Analyze and Write Individual Case Reports

According to Stake (1995), "There is no particular moment when data analysis begins. The analysis is a matter of giving meaning to first impressions as well as to final compilations" (p. 71). After the data were collected, the next step was qualitative data analysis. Initially, each case site was individually analyzed based on interviews, documents, archival data, and evidence. The following provides an understanding of the analysis of the collected data.

Questionnaires

Questionnaires were developed and distributed to determine the interview participants. The questionnaire contained demographic and historical informational questions, Likert scale measurements, and open-ended questions.

Open-ended questions on the questionnaire were analyzed by coding and theme creation based on the investigation of the research questions. All open-ended questions were interpreted through multi-cycle in vivo coding based on Saldaña' (2016) outline. Using the participant's own words, in vivo coding was used to heighten awareness of each participant's unique and individual circumstances. Cross themes were developed by combining all open-ended questionnaire data at each case site.

Interviews

In-depth data analysis of interviews focused on coding and theme creation was constructed on the investigation of the research questions. All interviews were audio recorded and transcribed verbatim. Identical to the process of the questionnaire coding, all interviews/focus groups were interpreted through multi-cycle codes, according to Saldaña (2016). Using the participant's own words, in vivo coding was used to have a heightened awareness of each participant's unique and individual circumstances. Cross themes were developed by combining all interview data at each case site through descriptive coding of the in vivo codes and, finally, pattern coding to identify patterns and frequency of the emerged themes.

Documents

Additionally, in-depth data analysis of collected documents focused on coding and theme creation based on the investigation of the research questions. All documents were interpreted through descriptive coding, consistent with Saldaña (2016). By summarizing the contents and topics located within documents and field notes, descriptive coding leads to a "categorized inventory, tubular account, summary, or index of the data's content" (Saldaña, 2016, p. 104). Specifically, Saldaña (2016) stated that by using descriptive coding to analyze basic topics, the researcher understands what is going on related to the study. In analyzing the documents within each case site to create an understanding of the impact of the opioid crisis and the school's preparedness, descriptive coding is an impactful method of coding to understand what is going on.

Archival Data

Archival data is a secondary source to analyze accruing trends and provide evidence of the phenomenon. This study documents and reviews data such as special education referrals and the percentage of students receiving special education services over the past few years. Overdose data about the district involved was collected through local law enforcement.

Considerations

Data analysis was identical within the three case studies, but access to the data at each case site varied minimally. The following steps were a cross-case analysis within each of these case sites.

Analysis, Interpretation, and Cross-Case Reports

The next step in analyzing the data was to combine the information collected from all three sites and complete a cross-case analysis and report. Once each case site was analyzed and an individual report was created, the next steps included drawing cross-case conclusions between all three case sites, including a collective analysis of results, development of policy and school implications, and concluding with a cross-case report.

Interview Coding Method

According to Stake, "Each researcher needs, through experience and reflection, to find the forms of analysis that work for him or her" (Stake, 1995, p. 77). All interviews in the three schools were coded in the same way. *The Coding Manual for Qualitative Researchers* by Saldaña (2016) was used to determine coding strategies. In all 29 interviews, three coding cycles were utilized – in vivo coding was the first cycle, followed by descriptive coding, and finally, pattern coding. Specific themes emerged after the three coding cycles, and codes were distributed in the coding categories. Additionally, categories were arranged by superordinate and subordinate arrangements to focus the investigation's parameters on finding the core and answering each specific research question. A select number of dominant themes emerged based on the research questions.

The coding cycle started with in vivo coding. After each interview was transcribed, each interview was read through three times, then coded line by line. A list of impactful words spoken by the participants was created from each interview and sorted into similar themes. To understand the process, the following examples of in vivo codes were pulled from five different participants' words during interviews:

- "Homeless population increasing and transiency increasing."
- "There is drug-related transiency because students move around missed school."
- "Kids are taken away from parents, or they go stay with others and miss school a lot."
- "Kids in and out of homes, double up in apartments, leading to missing school."
- "Sometimes, when foster care is involved, we do not see students again."

Next, descriptive coding was utilized using the participant's words collected through in vivo methods. By summarizing the contents and topics of interviews, descriptive coding led to a "categorized inventory, tubular account, summary, or index of the data's content" (Saldaña, 2016, p. 104). Specifically, Saldaña (2016) stated that by using descriptive coding to analyze basic topics, the researcher understands what is occurring in the study.

Similar quotes were then categorized together from all participants. Based on those five examples, I labeled the code descriptively as "transiency." All quotes that fell under transiency (the superordinate category) were grouped, then subordinate categories emerged on why the transiency was happening based on participants' insight. This was the second step in the descriptive process. The reason for transiency was then listed as follows:

Transiency

- Foster care
- Homelessness
- Parental instability

This process was continued through all the emerging themes. After in vivo coding and descriptive coding were complete, each interview theme was analyzed to find patterns and percentages created on how frequently the codes emerged in the combination of all interviews. If a code emerged 50% or more during the combined interviews, it became the dominant theme of the case.

Pattern coding was the third and final method used to make generalized conclusions between all three cases by highlighting similarities, differences, and frequencies.

According to Saldaña (2016), pattern coding identifies similarities, differences, frequency, sequence, correspondence, and causation within the themes and categories and establishes patterns. By interpreting similarities, differences, frequencies, sequences, correspondence, and causation within themes, the researcher can draw cross-case conclusions, develop policy implications, interpret the information collected, and uncover generalizations and conclusions between all three case sites.

Instrumentation and Validation Process

The research incorporated several processes to demonstrate the trustworthiness of the data analyzed, which supported the study's legitimacy. The processes included survey validation, triangulation of the findings, member checking, creating an audit trail, and maintaining a field journal.

The Validity of the Instrument

Although this was a qualitative study, a survey was used and shared to collect background data, qualitative evidence, and interview volunteers. The questionnaire's accuracy, reliability, and validity were measured through sample representatives, a team, and a focus group of content experts in various fields. Such fields include quantitative statistics, developmental psychology, sociology, criminology, human development, early childhood, and educational leadership.

Through convened meetings with the content expert focus group, an independent review of the tool was completed to determine the effectiveness, and the contents of the survey were validated. The researchers and content experts reviewed and collaborated on the survey's content, measurement tool, and wording.

In addition to the interdisciplinary team of content experts, the survey was distributed to a test group of representatives ($n = 63$) to validate the survey's wording, interpretation, and accuracy to confirm understanding. The representatives consisted of a population of classroom teachers, higher education professionals, school administrators, and other educators.

Triangulation

The validity of the research was measured through the triangulation of data collected within each case site. Salkind (2010) referred to triangulation as the practice of using multiple sources of data or various approaches to analyzing data to enhance the credibility of a research study. The triangulation incorporated and aligned multiple perspectives within this multiple-case study to create a more comprehensive understanding of the phenomenon. The data in the case study came from various sources and people. Teachers and various school and district administrators were interviewed, surveys were distributed, documents were collected, archival data was viewed, and member checking completed the process.

Member Checking

According to Creswell (2013), member checking, also known as participant or respondent validation, is a technique for exploring the credibility of researched results. In this study, the findings and data were shared with participants to check for accuracy and resonance with their experiences and preparedness. The member check confirmed the accuracy and validity of the results.

Audit Trail/Field Journal

A field journal was kept with notes and memoranda throughout the case-study investigation to track and bracket biases to minimize preconceptions and prejudices throughout the project. The journal also contained an audit trail as a transparent description of the steps, from starting a research project to developing and reporting findings. This journal served as a tool to separate personal thoughts from facts and findings, continuously tracking and bracketing biases. Considering past experiences, community involvement, the extended time at each research location, and the inherent nature of the research, tracking and bracketing through a field journal became necessary to minimize biases and increase objectivity.

Additional Research to Establish Validity

An additional study was conducted to prove external validity. The findings and procedure will be explained in Chapter 12.

Ethical Considerations

The research maintained ethical standards by ensuring the confidentiality of participants and school districts. All participation was voluntary and required informed consent. Participants were protected with anonymity and confidentiality, confirming no potential for harm. The school names were changed, and the participants' names were not released in the study. Pseudonyms are given to all participants in the field journal and named quotes. All necessary steps were taken to protect the rights and welfare of participants in all three studies discussed in this book. The three separate studies within this one overarching study were all approved through appropriate Internal Review Boards (IRBs), validating the adherence to ethical guidelines.

Bringing It All Together

This research study uses a multiple-case-study investigation that provided an in-depth, real-world analysis of three schools in three states located in opioid-crisis regions. The voice and lens of the educator was shared to fully grasp the perspective of the opioid epidemic from the view of the educator. Questionnaires, interviews, documents, archival data, and secondary observations were collected, coded, and analyzed. Furthermore, the research design collected data that purposefully created an understanding and raised awareness about the classroom impact of the opioid epidemic. If all or most cases provide similar results, there can be substantial support for developing a preliminary theory that describes a phenomenon (Eisenhardt, 1989). The data collection also highlighted the impact this crisis on education and recognized teachers' level of preparedness to teach students with potential cognitive, social, and behavioral implications that are evident as a direct result of the opioid epidemic.

References

Centers for Disease Control and Prevention. (2012). *Adverse childhood experiences (ACE) study.* National Center for Chronic Disease Prevention and Health Promotion. http://www.cdc.gov/ace/.

Centers for Disease Control and Prevention. (2015). Increases in drug and opioid overdose deaths–United States, 2000–2014. *Morbidity Mortality Weekly Report, 64*(50), 1–5.

Creswell, J. W. (2013). *Qualitative inquiry and research design: Choosing among five approaches* (3rd ed.). SAGE.

Eisenhardt, K. M. (1989). Building theories from case study research. *Academy of Management Review, 14*, 532–550.

Saldaña, J. (2016). *The coding manual for qualitative researchers* (3rd ed.). Sage.

Salkind, N. J. (2010). *Encyclopedia of research design.* Thousand Oaks, CA: SAGE Publications Ltd doi: 10.4135/9781412961288

Stake, R. E. (1995). *The art of case study research.* Sage.

Yin, R. K. (2018). *Case study research and applications: Design and methods* (6th ed.). Sage.

5 From Opioid Crisis to Classroom

The School Districts and Participants

> If we look at the saturation of the epidemic in the community it's a lot. We could come to school and find someone sleeping in our parking lot, passed out on a car, or passed out up in that grassy area (pointing). Just the other day, students were participating in an after-school event and witnessed a man overdose on the park bench across the street. One of the students had a phone and called 911. We see the adverse behaviors and it has such an impact on the children. My staff has clearly been affected, too. Last year I had two very young teachers admitted to the hospital with panic attacks, never had panic attacks before in their life. There are days that I'm sure some of them just don't want to come back and try this again. There are days that I don't want to come back and try this again. But I feel an obligation and I think that's what they do too. We are here for our babies.
>
> – Pat, New Hampshire Principal

The research unfolded across three public school communities in the heart of the Northeastern United States. These were not just any random schools – they were located in areas of the United States contending with the intense ramifications of the opioid crisis.

These districts were selected, using Centers for Disease Control (CDC) data, as having overdose rates threefold higher than compared to the rest of the nation. The CDC guidelines served as an indicator, guiding the search for areas where the fatal overdose toll exceeded 30 per 100,000 residents annually.

The next steps were to pinpoint exact cities and towns within these regions where the opioid crisis was profound. Law enforcement data was solicited in deciding an area to study. All locations had high drug-involved crime rates. In combination with law enforcement data and CDC overdose rates, the next step was to identify specific school districts located in major contributing areas.

Once districts were identified using the outlined criteria, and access was granted, a single school was identified within each city or town as the

DOI: 10.4324/9781003378204-6

focus of the case study. The particular school was identified through district administrator recommendations and access approval. Specifically, the three school districts investigated were in three states, Massachusetts, New Hampshire, and Maine.

There were 76 combined participants in this study out of 111 possible participants in the combined schools, totaling 68.4% total participation. There were 29 interviews conducted between 2018 and 2019. Of 29 interviews, 22 were in-person meetings, and seven were phone conferences. All face-to-face interviews occurred at the participants' schools. The survey was open and active from November 28, 2018, through February 4, 2019. There were 67 survey participants, and some participants participated in the survey and an interview.

The following percentages should be noted when calibrating all the teachers who participated in the research. There was a mix of experience levels throughout. Twenty-three percent (n = 18) of the survey and interview participants worked with students for less than five years, while 26% (n = 20) worked with students for 20+ years. Furthermore, 22% (n = 16) had 10–15 years of experience, 13% (n = 10) had 6–9 years of experience, 13% (n = 10) had 16–20 years of experience, and 3% (2) chose not to answer this question.

Here is a snapshot of each district. The school districts were very similar in size and student population.

Massachusetts School – Anderson Loop School

Anderson Loop School, situated in Massachusetts, stands among the numerous Pre-K to eighth-grade schools within its district. The district encompasses more than 5,000 students from a diverse range of seven racial and ethnic backgrounds. At the time under review, the district was identified as a high-needs urban area, housing a significant population of English Language Learners and students in the low socioeconomic bracket. Over 50% of the school's attendees were eligible for free or reduced-price lunch. The city also had a substantial immigrant community. The school prided itself on offering a wealth of extracurricular activities, food programs, and comprehensive before- and after-school care, catering to the children of the district. The majority of teachers held state licensure from Massachusetts, and most educators within the district boasted three or more years of teaching experience.

However, Anderson Loop School faced considerable challenges due to the opioid epidemic gripping the area. According to local law enforcement, the school is situated in a region that witnessed over 300 combined fatal/nonfatal opioid overdoses and more than 500 drug-related arrests in 2021 alone. A significant portion of the students attending Anderson Loop School resided in households directly affected by this epidemic.

Massachusetts Participants

With a total of 20 out of 32 possible participants from Massachusetts, there was 63% participation. All interviews were voluntary and had appropriate signed consent. Twenty people affiliated with Anderson Loop School provided this study with input and experiences.

During on-site visits to Anderson Loop School, seven participants, including principals, special education administrators, and teachers, were interviewed. Table 5.1 illustrates the seven participants' roles and type of interviews. Six interviews were face-to-face meetings, while one interview was a phone call. After seven interviews, saturation was achieved as the same themes, patterns, ideas, and opinions continued to emerge.

There was a range of knowledge and a number of years of teaching experience among the participants. Twenty-eight percent (n = 5) of the educators had one to five years of experience, while 28% (n = 5) had 20-plus years of experience. With participants' roles ranging from administration, teachers, and social workers to special educators, the epidemic's impact was captured through various lenses to triangulate the data. Regardless of the professionals interviewed or surveyed, it is evident through data collection that this opioid epidemic is causing a school crisis.

New Hampshire School – Cobbs Hill School

Nestled in New Hampshire, Cobbs Hill School is one of the district's schools, accommodating Pre-K to fifth-grade students. The district boasted a diverse population, hosting over 5,000 students of varied ethnicities due to the city's increasing immigration community. Offering many extracurricular activities, food programs, and pre- and post-school care, the school caters to the district's children. Over half of Cobbs Hill School's attendees were eligible for free or reduced-price lunches. The majority of the teachers held licensure from the state of New Hampshire, with a significant portion possessing three or more years of teaching experience within the district.

Table 5.1 Massachusetts Interview Participants

Massachusetts Interview Participant	*Role at MES*	*Type of Interview*
Massachusetts participant 1	Administrator	Telephone
Massachusetts participant 2	Administrator	In-person
Massachusetts participant 3	Teacher	In-person
Massachusetts participant 4	Teacher	In-person
Massachusetts participant 5	Special Education Teacher	In-person
Massachusetts participant 6	Teacher	In-person
Massachusetts participant 7	Administrator	In-person

The Cobbs Hill School found itself at the heart of the opioid crisis. Local law enforcement data revealed a distressing surge of over 35% in opioid overdoses within the vicinity between 2016 and 2022, resulting in more than 500 arrests related to opioid-related crimes. Schools in the vicinity grappled with the fallout of this epidemic, facing profound challenges.

New Hampshire Participants

There were 28 out of 38 possible participants, equating to a 74% participation rate at Cobbs Hill School. Twenty-six participants filled out the survey, and 12 participants were interviewed from administration, teachers, social workers, and consultants. All participation was voluntary and had appropriate signed consent. Table 5.2 illustrates the 12 interview participants' roles and type of interviews. Ten interviews were face-to-face in-person meetings, while two interviews were phone conferences. Two interview participants did not take the survey but were recommended to be interview participants by the school administrator; therefore, they were called and followed up with email communication. The two additional participants agreed to participate in the study and signed a participation consent. After 12 interviews, saturation was achieved as the same themes, patterns, ideas, and opinions continued to emerge.

There were 26 members of Cobbs Hill School who took the anonymous online survey. When combining all participants (interview and surveys), there was a variety of kindergarten through second-grade teachers, special educators, behavior and mental health support, instructional coaches, and administrators.

The experiences and professional responsibilities of the staff were diverse. Thirty-one percent ($n = 8$) of all participants had 20-plus years of experience,

Table 5.2 New Hampshire Interview Participants

New Hampshire Interview Participant	*Role at GES*	*Type of Interview*
New Hampshire participant 1	Administrator	In-person
New Hampshire participant 2	Behavior specialist	In-person
New Hampshire participant 3	Teacher	In-person
New Hampshire participant 4	Counselor	In-person
New Hampshire participant 5	Special education teacher	In-person
New Hampshire participant 6	Special education teacher	In-person
New Hampshire participant 7	Special education teacher	In-person
New Hampshire participant 8	Mental health provider	In-person
New Hampshire participant 9	Teacher	In-person
New Hampshire participant 10	Trauma consultant	Telephone
New Hampshire participant 11	Social Worker	In-person
New Hampshire participant 12	Instructional Coach	Telephone

while 19% (n = 5) had five or fewer years of experience working with students. The other participants had somewhere between 5 and 20 years of experience.

The participants included a diverse group of individuals because of the variety of expertise and years of experience. With various participants ranging from administration, teachers, special educators, social workers, behavior specialists, and consultants, the epidemic's impact was captured through various angles to triangulate the data collected. Viewpoints were captured through the diversity of the individual's experiences.

Maine School – Fox Hollow United School

Located in Maine, Fox Hollow United School is among numerous elementary schools in its district spanning from Pre-K to fifth grade. Embracing a diverse community, the school district encompasses over seven distinct races and ethnicities, reflecting a city with a significant immigrant population. Committed to holistic care, the school offers a variety of extracurricular activities, essential food programs, and comprehensive before- and after-school care catering to the district's children. More than half of the attending students benefit from free or reduced-price lunches.

The majority of Fox Hollow United School's educators are state-licensed, with a significant portion with three or more years of teaching experience.

According to the Opportunity Alliance Community Notes from 2018, Maine witnessed a distressing peak in opioid overdose deaths, reaching a staggering 418 in 2017 alone. Alarmingly, approximately 8% of all births in Maine were affected by Neonatal Abstinence Syndrome (NAS). Fox Hollow United School is at the heart of this crisis, embedded within a community struggling against this epidemic.

Fox Hollow United School has combined two school locations. The two schools were connected through their special education service model. Students with social-emotional and behavioral disabilities were taught at one site for academic and behavioral support that the main campus could not provide. Students transitioned between the school's unified arts or other classes. Still, for the most part, students were housed in the specific campus location to ensure their needs and related services were available. Both sites were investigated in an exploratory case study to develop an understanding of the impact the opioid epidemic was having on the school and the related community.

Both campuses of Fox Hollow United School participated in this case study. Kindergarten through second grade were the primary focus, with various participants ranging from a central office district administrator to school administrators, teachers, and social workers.

Maine Participants

With a total of 41 possible participants, there was a 68.2% participation rate. Twenty-eight people affiliated with Fox Hollow School gave input to this study. Participants volunteered for interviews in the survey, colleagues recommended participants, or people were recommended and asked to participate. All interviews were voluntary and had appropriate signed consent.

Ten participants were interviewed, from central office administrators to mental health providers, teachers, and school administrators. Table 5.3 illustrates the ten interview participants' roles and type of interviews. Six interviews were face-to-face meetings, while four interviews were phone calls. After ten interviews, saturation was achieved as the same themes, patterns, ideas, and opinions continued to emerge.

In combination with all the participants (interviews and surveys), there was a variety of kindergarten through second-grade teachers, special educators, behavior and mental health support, academic coaches, and administrators.

The participants bring a variety of expertise and several years of teaching experience: 26% ($n = 7$) of the participants had 10–15 years of experience, while 21% ($n = 5$) were in their first five years of teaching.

With participants ranging from central office administration, teachers, special educators, and social workers, the epidemic's impact was captured through numerous lenses to triangulate the data collected. Perspectives were entwined through multiple professionals who experienced the epidemic's impact from different views and expertise. All communications with professionals and data collected indicated a high state of concern with the opioid epidemic and its impact on the school.

Table 5.3 Maine Interview Participants

Maine Interview Participant	*Role*	*Type of Interview*
Maine participant 1	Administrator	In-person
Maine participant 2	Administrator	In-person
Maine participant 3	District administrator	Telephone
Maine participant 4	Teacher	In-person
Maine participant 5	Teacher	In-person
Maine participant 6	Teacher	In-person
Maine participant 7	Social worker	Telephone
Maine participant 8	Clinical social worker	In-person
Maine participant 9	Social worker	Telephone
Maine participant 10	Social worker	Telephone

Bringing It All Together

Although located in three different states within the United States, the three schools explored were similar in size, socioeconomic status, and needs. The three schools had many similarities. Specifically, the three school districts are located in urban areas with over seven races and ethnicities. According to the Massachusetts Department of Education's high-needs designation (2023), all three schools would be considered high-needs schools with large populations of students considered low-income, economically disadvantaged, English language learners, and students with disabilities.

Reference

Massachusetts Department of Education. (2023). *School districts and profiles: About the data.* https://profiles.doe.mass.edu/help/data.aspx?section=acct

Part 2

Understanding the Research Through Educators' Perspectives

The opioid crisis creates a complex atmosphere, profoundly impacting students, schools, and educators. In Part 2, educators' stories are shared to better understand the experiences, heartaches, and perspectives of those working in schools located in opioid epicenters. The stories vividly portray teachers' emotional strain and unwavering dedication amid the challenging landscape. Part 2 of the book includes Chapters 6–10. It explores the daunting student challenges educators face, such as exposure to countless adverse childhood experiences, homelessness, transiency, inadequate responses from the Department of Youth Services, and parental instability, among others. Despite initiatives by school districts, teachers express a sense of unpreparedness in their schools, emphasizing the lack of professional development and resources. This part highlights powerful quotes and unforgettable stories of our devoted educators working in crisis areas. Part 2 also shares entries from the field journals to create additional understanding of experiences and observations while on location.

DOI: 10.4324/9781003378204-7

6 Educators Share Stories of Student's Household and Environmental Opioid Exposures and Experiences

Week 5 Reflection from the Field Journal:

This is my fifth-week visiting schools. My days are full of interviewing educators, analyzing data such as special education trends, collecting professional development documents, interacting with law enforcement agencies, and immersing myself in the school environment. I spent hours in teacher's rooms and administrative offices, getting to know the dedicated educators and understanding the intricacies of the day-to-day operation.

Being physically present in these schools allowed me to witness firsthand the profound impact of the opioid crisis on the community. During this period, I observed distressing incidents, such as two men overdosing outside the school, visible through the window. Additionally, I encountered many individuals affected by the crisis, including waking up a gentleman sleeping outside the school entrance and learning the protocols to remove hazardous items like used needles, condoms, and empty glass bottles from school playgrounds.

Since I am well into my second month, I need to take a moment to reflect. I find myself thinking about one of the young teacher's quotes, "We are not taught this stuff in teacher prep!" How do you prepare future teachers for parents insisting on bringing pet squirrels into the school, students who witnessed a parent's murder, kindergartners playing with Barbies and pretending to flush drugs down the toilet when "Ken the Cop" arrives, and second graders who can explain the process to boot up heroin? I do not have answers, but we need to figure out solutions to address the population of children who come to school with the weight of unimaginable trauma and support the teachers who are witnessing such traumas.

These experiences were deeply moving and opened my eyes to the harsh realities faced by communities grappling with this public health emergency. It became evident that the crisis was no longer confined outside school walls; its repercussions were felt within the educational setting, affecting everyone – individuals of all ages from kindergarten students to administrators.

DOI: 10.4324/9781003378204-8

> Engaging directly with educators and stakeholders while immersing myself in the school, community, and environment provided a unique perspective. It went way beyond just data analysis, offering a profound understanding of the human toll and daily challenges faced by those affected by the opioid crisis.

The collected evidence and data indicated that drug-related activities in the environment significantly affect three schools and their classrooms. Interviews with participants unveiled that students' exposure to opioid-related activities profoundly and swiftly impacts both the classroom and the overall school environment due to its pervasive and continuous nature. Twenty-nine participants from all three schools were interviewed for this study. Opioid exposure was a coded theme that emerged within 100% ($N = 29$) of the interview participants. Other central patterns and codes associated with the exposure that emerged from the interviews were student behaviors 100% ($N = 29$) and parent and family instability 100% ($N = 29$). Also notable, in the calibration of the 67 survey results, the central themes that stemmed from exposure were student neglect 93% ($n = 62$), family instability 87% ($n = 58$), and involvement with the Department of Youth Services 79% ($n = 53$). These themes are briefly mentioned in this chapter and will be revisited.

The influence of opioid exposure, whether through residing in a household, neighborhood, or environment affected by the opioid crisis, directly affects schools within these regions experiencing the crisis.

The impact is tangible and widespread across all three areas, delineated by each school's unique circumstances. Educators interviewed shared first-hand experiences and narratives that vividly illustrate the toll of the opioid crisis on their schools. These accounts, conveyed through the educators' voices, carry poignant emotions and vividly articulate the profound effects witnessed within their educational settings.

Cobbs Hill School, New Hampshire

In New Hampshire, 38 educators qualified to participate in the study. Of the 38 participants, 28 agreed to participate, equating to a 74% participation rate.

At Cobbs Hill School in New Hampshire, opioid exposure was the most discussed theme among the 12 interview participants. Of the interview participants, 100% ($N = 12$) mentioned students' opioid-related exposure, and 69% ($n = 18$) of survey participants had students in their class who they confirmed were currently impacted by the opioid epidemic. Reoccurring coded themes that evolved from surveys and interviews from the New Hampshire educators included topics such as the normalcy of drug activity seen in their students' behaviors, actions, and imaginary play, the increased perception and knowledge that more and more students are born addicted to opioids, parental instability, and parental behaviors. Students are exposed to opioid abuse through family drug use, witnessing opioid-related crimes and opioid overdoses, and drug activity in the environment around the school. According to participants, young students normalized the drug culture and verbally and physically reenacted drug use behaviors on school grounds. Through exposure and experiences, the opioid use and exposure for the children of Cobbs Hill School was typical, regular, and readily evident. As a New Hampshire Behavior Specialist explained:

> We have a huge number of students directly impacted by the epidemic here. Our kids know way too much. They know what different substances look like, they know street names, they have been held at gunpoint over a drug deal gone wrong, and they have watched their parents and guardians inject heroin. They are taken out of their homes because of this epidemic. I would say that every single child in our school has experienced some type of trauma.

According to New Hampshire educators working at Cobbs Hill School, students' exposure impacts the school and learning environment. During the duration of the research, different situations were observed. For example, one day, a handful of second-grade students were caught in the bathroom snorting, selling, and marketing packets of Crystal Light, pretending it was a drug. Four interview participants shared the story during interviews because it happened on one of the weeks spent at the school. The situation was mentioned in all four interviews to explain how normalized and accepted drug behavior is in the community and how the exposure is very evident within the schools.

The quotes and explanations of the normalcy of drug activity and behaviors were remarkable. For example, a second-grade teacher said, "My students could not tell you what an aquarium is, but they can explain the process to boot up heroin." According to a K-2 special education teacher:

> These kids come in here and start talking about people using drugs, their parents using drugs, and all the people in their building that OD'd. When we see an ambulance go by these kids are like, "Oh, I bet someone OD'd." That is their first go to. I am thinking of a car accident, right? They think OD.

Participants discussed how exposure to the epidemic surrounds the school, and students talk about it because it is normalized in their lives.

A second-grade teacher explained that the community surrounding the school is "full of violence and many drugs. Drugs and violence lead to the neglect of our students." According to educators, the environment most children of Cobbs Hill School are exposed to is full of crime, drugs, and violence.

The principal recounted how students participating in an after-school event witnessed a man overdose on the park bench across the street. One of the students had a phone and called 911. The administrator explained the problem's proximity on school grounds: "we could come to school and find someone sleeping in our parking lot, passed out on the car, or up in that grassy area." In addition to the administrator's concerns, two teachers mentioned that drug activity was occurring around the school; hypodermic needles were found near or on the school playground and grounds.

According to existing research, students at Cobbs Hill School have witnessed traumatizing events that would impact learning and focus. Within the 12 interviews, various duplicated and confirming stories were mentioned. According to a first-grade teacher, "I do not know how my six-year-old processes seeing her mom stick needles in her arms, the whole situation we are dealing with is heartbreaking." Specifically, students at Cobbs Hill School have witnessed an overdose death of a parent. A second grader found her uncle deceased in a tub, children have had guns held to their heads in a dispute over drug money, and parents have trafficked their children for money to feed their addiction. A counselor explained:

> Students are so aware of the drugs out there, and they see things; they see parents doing them, family members doing them. I have had several kids that have witnessed overdoses in their homes. And I have had other students the brunt of people coming into their homes and holding them at gunpoint because people living in their home owed drug dealer's money.

Additionally, children are being pulled from their homes overnight by police or the Department of Youth Services (DYS) and, according to participants, come to school the next day exhausted. Two participants shared a story about "parents taking their children to doctors' appointments high on heroin and the children watching them get arrested in their pediatrician's office." As an administrator said, "You can imagine they are not learning their multiplication tables, right? There is a reason for that. There is a reason for that, right?" Academic success was hardly a topic of any of the interviews – educators continuously mentioned that there were many more critical issues to resolve before focusing on increasing academic success rates.

In addition to opioid use exposure, educators at Cobbs Hill School show concern about the students who were possibly born exposed to opioids and had Neonatal Abstinence Syndrome (NAS). The following section describes the educator's challenges and perspectives.

Neonatal Abstinence Syndrome

New Hampshire educators at Cobbs Hill School repeatedly mentioned the increased number of children in their classes or on their special education caseloads who were born addicted to opioids. Specifically, 75% ($n = 9$) of the interview participants mentioned that they were concerned about the documented amount and increased numbers of children born with NAS. According to survey participants, 56% ($N = 14$) of the educators had a student in their class who was confirmed to be born with NAS either through Individualized Education Program (IEP) documentation or through family/guardian communication.

Three New Hampshire special educators interviewed at Cobbs Hill School mentioned such examples. According to one special education teacher, "We had so many kids that were born addicted. We are seeing those students not only with learning difficulties but so many other difficulties." A kindergarten teacher and social worker emphasized that the number of children exposed to "opioids *in utero*" is rapidly growing in the community. According to another teacher, "Opioids have affected our school severely. We not only have many families with at least one parent addicted, we have many students that were born addicted." One teacher added, "I have children in my class that were born addicted, kids that parents know were born addicted, and nothing has been done for them, and they are delayed." In addition to the teachers, the principal added that NAS births are a frequent discussion in IEP meetings: "we see a lot of it. I sit in our student's IEP meetings, and I hear about how many days they as a baby were in the hospital coming down from their high and then need treatment." According to educators, students born prenatally exposed to opioids, exposure to opioid use at home and in the community, and other associated traumatizing events can directly impact the classroom. Special educators and administrators explained that there is also confusion about the IEP disability category for students with cognitive and emotional delays due to drug exposure – a possible area for future research.

Parental and Home Instability

Another coded theme that emerged in the interviews at Cobbs Hill School was the concern with parental instability. Specifically, parental instability was mentioned by 100% ($N = 12$) of New Hampshire educators interviewed. Parental instability includes grandparents raising children because parents are unable to due to the consequences of addiction. When viewing the family through the educators' lens, addiction results in the instability of the home. Children are transitioning from one house to another, in and out of foster care, and grandparents are raising children.

According to a first-grade teacher:

> Many kids live in families with active use, but many of our children live with extended family members. They could be living with an aunt or a grandparent because of a parent's addiction, or parents are incarcerated because of drugs.

According to the Cobbs Hill principal:

> The number of grandparents that are raising children in this building is extraordinary. We have one grandparent. The little boy is in second grade and was born with addicted. Mother was addicted, and now she's incarcerated, so the grandmother has him and he's very behaviorally involved. She, grandma also has her son's two children in addition for the same issue. Drugs. And in that same apartment, there's another family that attends school here where the grandmother is the custodian of the children, and they all live together and take care of all those kids together.

Teachers mentioned that grandparents raising children in homes is the norm. A kindergarten teacher noted that students think that it is odd not to be raised by a grandmother. Out of a class of 22, this teacher had five grandparents raising her students, two siblings in their early 20s raising siblings, and a few active and open foster care situations. In this kindergarten class, she confirmed that 9 out of 22 students were not living with mom or dad. The teacher was then asked why she thought her class was dealing with such an influx of children raised by grandparents, and she confirmed that half of those were confirmed drug-related, and she suspected that the other half were likely related to drugs as well.

On a positive note, a kindergarten teacher applauded a grandparent for positive changes in her student. According to the kindergarten teacher:

> The principal informed the teacher of the change in living arrangements, and I saw a huge difference, but for the better, because he was with grandma. He was coming in clean. He had new clothes on. You could tell he was eating. He didn't look like he hadn't showered in a week. He was smiling, because I think he got a good night's sleep, and he was really trying to please me and do his job. I think that was because of the support he was getting at home. But unfortunately, I knew the day that he went back to mom, because everything went back to how it was, and he's still back with mom. It is so sad. All his parents had to do was pass a drug test

> to get custody back. We all know she is still on drugs, but unfortunately, it takes a crisis.

Parental instability is a theme that emerged as causing anxiety in students at Cobbs Hill School. Sometimes students needed to find out who would be watching them each day. In addition to the instability, Cobbs Hill School has to determine the best way to maneuver parental behaviors and aggressions on location at the school.

Parents' Behaviors

Parental behavior was a theme throughout the interviews at Cobbs Hill School. Of the New Hampshire educators interviewed, 83% (n = 10) mentioned parental behaviors. It should be noted that none of the interview questions specifically asked about the parent's behaviors. This was an unexpected theme that emerged within the interviews. Educators described parents as guarded, secretive, disengaged, aggressive, addicted, and neglectful.

Specifically, teachers were concerned that parents were coming into school under the influence. A special education teacher expressed concern that parents were high coming to IEP meetings. She wondered if they could legally sign off on special education services under the influence.

The principal added a few stories that highlighted the behaviors of parents under the influence on school grounds that they had to deal with:

> We had a father arrested in the lobby who came in high as a kite. I came into the lobby and immediately asked my secretary to call 911 and we put the building in lockdown. The police walked through the door, they took one look at him and put him face down on the floor and handcuffed him and took him away.

The principal continued with another story:

> I had an incident with a parent, where the parent was screaming in my face, again, the F word, and other things. And the next day the fourth grader came to see me on his own and said, I'm really sorry about my dad.

And another added:

> We've had parents engage each other physically on the property. There's a food pantry here on Saturdays so the fight started at the food pantry, and then the Monday following, the two women are outside my window here, engaged, physically engaged with each other. The windows are

> open, the profanity is flying. It's just a, the boundaries, it's a consistent issue with lack of boundaries. Both these women are mothers and known heroin abusers.

The final story specific to parental behavior almost led to another visit by local law enforcement:

> A mom came to do the volunteer to pop popcorn last week and the tee shirt said, one, two, three, fuck you. On the back. So, I went out in the lobby and I said to her, ma'am, you either have to go turn that inside out in the bathroom, put your coat on, or you need to leave. She fought me with the freedom of speech. She ended up leaving but I was about to call the police. Sure enough, she was high.

The principal concluded by explaining, "Parent behavior is a problem. Some parents are consistently intoxicated or under the influence that cannot come on the property because they have threatened me or others on the property."

A few teachers explained that the parents do not want anyone in their homes because of fear of exposure to drug activity. Teachers advocate and find outside community resources to help families but are not utilizing them because of fear of exposure. According to teachers, parents do not approve administration and often outside resources that teachers advocate for their students. They are reluctant for their children to receive outside therapy or home visits. Teachers are also concerned that they are ill-prepared to deal with the parents, which can be frightening and stressful. Consequently, due to the epidemic, parental behaviors impact teachers and lead to teacher stress, burnout, and secondary trauma. Secondary teacher trauma will be addressed in Chapter 8.

New Hampshire educators shared their stories and concern about the normalcy of drug exposure, the increase of students born addicted, and the consequences of parental instability and behaviors. The following section takes a deep dive into similar effects of exposure at Main Fox Hollow United School.

Fox Hollow United School, Maine

In Maine, 41 educators qualified to participate in the study, and out of the 41 participants, 28 agreed to participate, equating to a 68% participation rate.

Like students attending Cobbs Hill School in New Hampshire, students at Fox Hollow School in Maine were exposed to drug activity through their experiences at home, in their neighborhood, and in proximity to the school. One of the notable differences between the teacher's perspectives in Maine versus New Hampshire was the amount of drug activity witnessed from the seats of the schools in Maine. Educator interviews revealed that environmental factors such as exposure, family drug use, the vicinity of drug activity, poverty, homelessness, parental fluctuation, born with NAS, neglect, and instability are impacting the classroom. Specifically, 100% (N = 10) of those interviewed mentioned student exposure to drug activity, homelessness, parental instability, and parent behaviors, while 90% (n = 9) mentioned unmet basic needs. Here are the calibrated stories and the lens of the opioid crisis shared by Maine educators with a focus on exposure, parental instability, and behaviors.

Opioid Exposure at Home and in the Community

Through interviews and surveys, Maine educators shared that students have witnessed parents, strangers, and other family members use drugs, overdose, and die from opiate abuse. According to a social worker at Fox Hollow United, "The epidemic is having a direct impact on the classroom and the school. Students are experiencing deaths of parents, family members, and adult friends of families." Another social worker added, "I had a student who witnessed their mom trying to be resuscitated after an overdose. She did not make it." These situations were constant and prevalent, impacting the classrooms and school.

Consequently, teachers felt the same as social workers. One teacher added:

> The opioid epidemic is impacting my classroom in the sense that the kids are dealing with a parent that is addicted. I had one kid last year. One parent was using, and one parent was not. The using parent was in and out, but the dad was a good parent but just could keep the mom out of the house. It was heartbreaking. That student was put in foster care, because Mom kept coming back.

Another teacher explained, "All of my students are affected by the opioid epidemic in one way or another, including myself. The majority of my students have a parent who is either in active addiction or has used in the past."

In addition to watching parents and family members use drugs, students at Fox Hollow United were exposed to drugs in their community and environment. Interview participants linked community drug exposure to classroom impact. A second-grade teacher explained:

> Even if these kids don't deal with it in their immediate household, they are living in an area or neighborhood that they are being exposed to it everywhere. They see stuff, hear stuff, and know bad stuff is happening around them all the time, and they come to school in crisis.

A social worker explained that students cannot even escape by going to local facilities: "The kids can go to the local YMCA, but unfortunately, there is no escape because people are doing drugs in that building, too." Exposure to opioid abuse and environmental factors were frequently identified within the body of each interview as having a direct impact on the school.

Educators also revealed that the conditions and exposure students had at school directly impacted learning. The proximity of homeless shelters that surround the school attracted a culture of drug and drug activity. A clinical social worker described the surroundings of Fox Hollow United as an abundance of "floridly psychotic, drug-addicted, and then the people that are preying on those people." Looking out the windows, walking to the bus, and playing in the playground, students watched people surrounding the school participate in such activities.

A teacher added, "[T]he opioid epidemic is constantly affecting my classroom. My students are not only exposed to drug abuse in their homes but right outside the windows of their school."

Additionally, another social worker expressed concern for not only the students but also the teachers, staff, and parents who are exposed to the environment:

> Students are being schooled in areas in which students, parents, teachers, and staff have to walk over used needles in the streets and sidewalks to get to school. Students are watching people shoot up in their cars outside the classrooms and pass out. People urinate outside classroom windows. . . . Middle schoolers used to put signs in the window that would say "this is a school don't smoke or whatever here" "this is a school, don't urinate here." Within the square block of the school . . . we were losing one person a day to a heroin overdose.

An administrator who worked in the building shared the same concerns as the two social workers and the teacher, highlighting that the school environment was having a direct impact on the school:

> Look outside this window! This is a direct impact. We all see adults using and dealing all day long. See that window? Somebody leaves drugs on that window, then somebody else comes and picks it up. I see people right there (pointing outside office window) shooting up heroin. Unfortunately, our young children here are watching this too.

One hundred percent of the Maine educators interviewed ($N = 10$) at Fox Hollow United revealed stories that described students directly impacted by the epidemic through exposure from their family, community, and proximity to the school.

Parental Instability and Parents' Behaviors

Like New Hampshire, Maine educators interviewed and surveyed described parents in active addiction as disengaged, unreachable, unstable, aggressive, and on the move. Of the total number of participants, 92% (n = 25) mentioned that students live with relatives other than their parents due to addiction. Numerous concerns about parents' recovery and relapse cycles caused overwhelming anxiety in the Fox Hollow School students. Like Cobbs Hill School, grandparents, aunts, and foster families were raising children.

According to the principal at Fox Hollow:

> Parents are good for a while, they're sober for a while, they're not, and then they are sober for a while, and again they're not. Kids learn not to be able to depend on anything. You know, so, "Oh, Mom's being really great now. Everything is great at home, uh oh, it's back." So, they can never relax and depend on their parents, and I think that's really damaging going forward in their life.

Additionally, there were many active Department of Family Service open cases at Fox Hollow. A teacher explained the instability of a parent, "The kids know there were drugs involved, and eventually, kids get taken out and put in foster care, but it usually takes a crisis." She went on to explain the struggles of parental behaviors.

I know that it's affecting my classroom in the sense that they're kids all the time who are dealing with a parent that are on drugs. The biggest impact is that kids leave and they're taken away. Sometimes we have kids that leave the school and put in foster care, or they have to go stay with somebody else. I've done many a conference where parents come in, and you just know, they are high and you have to report it. These kids are constantly in and out of their homes. There is no stability.

Parental behavior was also inappropriate on school grounds. An administrator explained:

> Parents get escalated very quickly. Yelling, screaming, arguing for no reason. And you just have to take it and wait until they're done and then say your point. Then they come around. It's almost like they're a child still, and you just let them have their tantrum.

As an unintended parallel finding between the three case studies and schools, parental behaviors and instability were prominent themes throughout the interview. It was a theme worth mentioning since it was mentioned in all three locations across all three states. Additionally, the Massachusetts Anderson Loop School had similar concerns regarding opioid exposure. Parental behaviors was another unintended suggested finding that would benefit from further investigation as educators may need tools, resources, trainings and additional skills to navigate.

Anderson Loop School, Massachusetts

In Massachusetts, 32 educators qualified to participate in the study. Of the 32 participants, 20 agreed to participate, equating to a 63% participation rate.

Similar to New Hampshire and Maine, participating Massachusetts educators expressed concern that many students at the Anderson Loop School were exposed to drug activity through their experiences at home. Interviews and survey results of the 20 participants revealed that environmental factors such as exposure, family drug use, poverty, homelessness, parental fluctuation, born addicted, neglect, and instability were impacting the classroom. Specifically, out of the seven participants interviewed, 100% mentioned student exposure, neglect, parent instability, and parent behaviors, while six of the seven educators said household crime. According to survey results, 82% ($n = 16$) reported that students in their classrooms have been removed from their homes because of household addiction, and 91% ($n = 18$) reported that students were neglected because of household addiction.

All of the interviewed educators believed that outside opioid exposure directly impacts the classroom. According to the educators, students at the Anderson Loop School are exposed by watching their parents engage in drug activity and are frequently exposed to related crime. Incarcerated parents and opioid use exposure were prominent themes throughout the interviews as impacting the classroom. In addition to exposure, survey results report that neglect and basic needs being unmet were a result of exposure.

Massachusetts educators shared the prominent themes of exposure and crime, parental instability, and behaviors. Massachusetts educators mentioned incarceration, crime, murder, and prostitution more than the participants in New Hampshire and Maine, making one wonder if student exposure to serious crime is more prevalent in Massachusetts than in New Hampshire and Maine. Massachusetts educators mentioned crime and incarceration frequently, which is noteworthy and an area for possible further investigations.

Exposure and Crime

Massachusetts teachers and administrators explained situations that their students had witnessed. The interviews revealed that numerous students witnessed an overdose death of a parent, lived in homes under the suspicion of drug deals, had parents incarcerated because of drugs, or watched adults inject drugs. This quote shared by the assistant principal sums up many interview themes discussed by the Massachusetts educators.

> The impact of the opioid epidemic is intense and is seen here through extreme behaviors. Kids are clearly living with trauma. Many kindergartners this year that have come in from situations where you can see the direct effect of a mother or father who's incarcerated, mother and father who are addicts, kindergartners who have come in under the care of other relatives that have communicated to us that addiction is part of the issue. Or already part of the foster care program, or under state custody. And we've seen a real influx this year in not just troublesome, problematic behaviors, but very extreme behaviors from children who are clearly in crisis from the trauma of dealing with this epidemic in their everyday lives.

Due to the trauma of the epidemic, students are suffering. For example, a second-grade student watched her mother fatally overdose on heroin. The second-grade teacher explained the situation and the impact: "we had a student whose mother overdosed, and the second grader, the daughter, was the one who found her mother. Can you imagine the impact?"

Another teacher added:

> I had a student that used to get locked in a closet all night long so mom could go out and prostitute to make money for drugs. He knows this and he talks about it. He used to be kept in a closet. He is emotionally needy and not needy at the same time. He wants to hug but then he wants to hate you. He doesn't know what it means to have a relationship with other people. His mom is now dead, and he will tell you his mom died because she did too many drugs.

All seven interviewed educators had a story that explained a tragic situation that directly impacted students in the classroom. According to participants, because of the situations the students were exposed to, students were coming to school without necessities and with undeniable evidence of neglect.

Parental Instability and Parents' Behaviors

The Massachusetts educators who were interviewed explained that parental instability is causing stress and anxiety to the students of the Anderson Loop School. Students continually move from one caregiver to the other, from one foster home to another. According to educators the unknown – not knowing whom the child is going home to or where the child will end up each day – is impacting their students focus, learn, and ability to relax causing stress for their students throughout the day.

According to the assistant principal:

> We have students who are having a really difficult time with their foster placement. Kids had been removed from drug abuse in the home and the

> kids are struggling to get acclimated to a new foster family. These kids are longing for a relationship with their biological parents. They may or may not understand the mechanisms at work here. And then we also have children who have been removed from really challenging situations that the state has custody and can't find foster care. So we have kids who are kind of bouncing back and forth between different homes, that have been removed from homes due to drug abuse and they are bouncing back and forth between temporary foster homes and group homes and it's just created a lot of instability in not only kids lives, but also in our ability to provide a consistent system of support for them because of how unstable their lives are.

As a teacher explained, "it is hard to worry if students are listening to my math lesson when they are wondering if their mom is safe and will still be home when they leave school." The following quotes describe the impact of parental instability.

According to a second-grade teacher:

> Mom got kicked out. Mom would come back. Grandma said she was being bad again. Oh she's back again. Just back and forth, and back and forth. You know, I could tell the minute that kid walked in my classroom if mom was back in the picture or if mom had been kicked back out again. That's really hard to watch. Why can't I worry about this kid paying attention to my math lesson when she wants to know, "Is my mother still living with me? Is my mother still safe?" That sort of thing.

A K-2 special education teacher added:

> I have a number of students, in second grade, where the students have lived with grandparents or an aunt or uncle, usually an aunt. People other than the parents. I have somebody who's in foster care. Mom is trying to get back custody. I know there are obstacles to that and that's a situation and I suspect a substance abuse problem where the foster mom is very on top of things, very organized, student comes to school regularly, looking great, and when there's a visit with mom, things seem to go very poorly.

A first-grade teacher had a similar story:

> A first grader was removed from her mother because her mother was battling a heroin addiction. . . . I think she did go to jail for drug related offenses. But the grandmother has communicated to us that she's been battling addiction. The mother is still allowed supervised visits. And so, the grandparents are trying to manage what's best for the child, but also

> trying to manage maintaining a relationship with the mom and the child is kind of caught in the middle and you can see that she's been in chaos. The little girl is in chaos.

In addition to the parental instability, parental behavior was causing a problem at Anderson Loop School. According to Massachusetts teachers, parents were coming to school and sometimes assaulting administrators, leading to evacuations and lockdowns. Furthermore, many participants mentioned that parents were coming to school projecting odd behaviors. For example, a woman came to school to pick up her children numerous times with her two pet squirrels, Julia and Peanut, on a leash, in her blouse, and resting on her shoulder.

The school principal was one of the four participants who mentioned a story involving the parent and pet squirrel:

> We have a mum who we strongly suspect is using drugs. And this particular family decided to take it upon themselves to start having pet squirrels in the home. And they get the squirrels by capturing them. Mum would sneak the squirrel into school by keeping the squirrel in her blouse, in her shirt. We had a parent meeting in the conference room with the squirrel. Mom had it under her shirt and it was freaking us out. It was ridiculous. The squirrel actually came up out of her shirt, and crawled up and was sitting on her head. And she had it on a leash. It was insane. I was beside myself. I think I was hyperventilating. But this was totally normal to her. On a different occasion, she came in when the child had torn apart the classroom and was making animal noises and grunting. And she came in with the squirrel. The squirrel, again, was on a leash. She was trying to help the child pick up the classroom and the squirrel's running around the classroom making more of a ruckus. It was just. . . . It was crazy. It was mind-boggling. And then you wonder, did the squirrel bite the child? What is happening in this household?

Another story shared by an administrator was about a father who went to an IEP meeting and was preoccupied with discussing Hitler and other dark historical events rather than their child's progress. Nothing could get the father back on track to discuss his child. Instead, he quickly changed moods, having a swearing screaming fit out of nowhere, screaming at the administrators and teachers involved. Most instances of odd behaviors were parents who were known drug users. This particular situation was a known drug user in the district.

According to the educators interviewed, teachers were nervous because they were exposed to these behaviors. One teacher mentioned, "We are not taught this stuff in teacher prep." As described by an administrator, parent behaviors "are really escalating – swearing and the screaming to actual physical assault. In fact, we have had two physical assaults this year on administration."

According to interview participants, parent instability and behaviors were having a direct impact on the classroom. Parents were adding to the stress of the day, not just concerning children but the teachers, staff, and administration as well. Parental behaviors and instability were unintentional findings worth mentioning and could benefit from further investigations in the future.

Similar to New Hampshire and Maine, Massachusetts educators had concerns that exposure, parental instability, and parent behaviors impacting school day-to-day operations.

Bringing It All Together

By investigating into educators' perspectives and understanding their detailed quotes, a profound understanding emerges regarding their perception of how the opioid epidemic is shaping their schools and classrooms. The evidence and gathered data emphasize that the presence of drug activity in the environment directly affects all three schools and their classroom dynamics.

Participants in the interviews highlighted how students' exposure to opioid-related activities significantly and abruptly disrupted both the classroom environment and the overall school atmosphere due to its pervasive and all-encompassing nature. Notably, educators across the three schools expressed worries regarding exposure, parental instability, and the impact of parents' behaviors within the school setting.

Subsequent chapters will delve deeper into exploring the ramifications of such exposure, shedding light on the effects of home instability and environmental influences on attendance rates, secondary trauma experienced by teachers, and academic achievements.

7 Navigating the Ripple Effects

Opioid Epidemic's Impact on Student Transiency, Homelessness, and Attendance

Thoughts from the Field Journal:

As I reside in schools, the disparities in resources become strikingly apparent. While one school has a McKinney-Vento guidance counselor dedicated to supporting and monitoring homeless students, the second school has a staff member in charge of monitoring students under the McKinney-Vento law as an added role in their many administrative priorities, and the third school lacks knowledge of who's responsible for monitoring homeless populations and McKinney-Vento initiatives. Their reasoning? A few participants told me that their funds are channeled into statewide assessment improvements, leaving no room for what they consider a non-academic hire. They claim ignorance, blaming top-down prioritized initiatives focusing on assessments rather than the needs of students.

Furthermore, one school stands out with a six-person dedicated attendance team committed to locating missing students daily, diligently scouring the city for any no-shows. This contrasts with another district where a single attendance resource officer oversees over 6,000 students. The disparities between districts are overwhelming, highlighting the need for standardized procedures, especially in schools lacking vital resources.

Contemplating these discrepancies, I'm struck by the inequalities and the profound impact that uniform processes could have on these underserved schools. Yet, considering the immense financial and resource implications of implementing such consistent procedures across the entirety of the United States, I wonder where and how to initiate such changes.

The effects of transiency, homelessness, and poverty pose significant challenges for educators in schools located in regions affected by the opioid crisis. Specifically, these issues have a substantial impact on attendance. Educators have shared their firsthand experiences and perspectives on how transiency, homelessness, and poverty affect attendance, consequently affecting the overall environment, achievements, and quest for resources and student

DOI: 10.4324/9781003378204-9

support – all of which significantly impact the functions of their schools and classrooms.

When considering the overarching themes across these schools, factors like student homelessness, transiency, poverty, neglect, unstable home environments, and the instability of parents or guardians directly affect attendance rates. Teachers attribute household addiction as the primary cause behind the interconnected problems of poverty, homelessness, and transiency, leading students to move between schools, districts, states, homeless shelters, and various guardians, such as grandparents, aunts, uncles, and cousins. This constant movement results in irregular school attendance, and some students become lost within the educational system. As reported by participants in the study, these hardships significantly impact schools and the day-to-day operations.

In the interview data, 28 out of the 29 (97%) educators mentioned transiency and homelessness as significantly impacting the classroom or the school. Additionally, of the 67 survey participants, 57 (85%) participants experienced a situation that resulted in a student's removal from the home because of a drug-related situation, 58 (87%) participants have students living with a relative because of household addiction, and 45 (67%) survey participants have students with open cases with the departments of youth services. In combination, 87% (n = 58) of all participants felt that the challenges of living in a home with active addiction impacted attendance and the day-to-day operations of the school.

Furthermore, educators highlighted that students affected by the opioid epidemic experience constant housing fluctuations, leading to significant instability and anxiety in the students who are constantly experiencing the unknown. Teachers noted the grave challenges in maintaining regular routines, offering additional assistance, managing behavioral referrals, providing special education evaluations, following through with intervetion referrals, and implementing ongoing initiatives. For instance, when students are referred for an evaluation for possible special education services and stop attending school before the evaluation concludes, evaluations are incomplete, and students are delayed in receiving appropriate special education services.

The transient nature of student attendance emerged as the predominant theme across the three schools discussed. Consistent conversations among these schools revolved around the frequent flux of students, their enrollment and withdrawal patterns, and the concerns arising when students abruptly stop attending classes only to reappear weeks or months later.

An overview of each school follows using quotes from educators to narrate and explain the situations better to understand their experiences and perspectives through their lens.

Cobbs Hill School, New Hampshire

Homelessness, poverty, and transiency frequently emerged from the New Hampshire interviews when asked, "How does the opioid epidemic impact your classroom/school?" New Hampshire educators credited the opioid crisis and drug abuse for much of the homelessness and transient students living in poverty. They explained that the inconsistency of student attendance and instability of the student's living conditions caused unpredictable student behaviors and impacted the consistency of the classroom.

An administrator explained that "many parents can barely take care of themselves, so they are obviously not taking care of their children, leading to homelessness. The number of people doubled up in this community because losing their homes to addiction is rampant."

The principal of Cobbs Hill explained her pleas to get the students to school despite parental turmoil associated with the epidemic:

> We have a huge issue with tardiness, and we're working on that. I bought a bunch of alarm clocks for kids to help them be independent. But again, think about it. It's important. My kids got out of bed and went to school because I made sure that they did that, but if your life is in turmoil for whatever reason, most likely connected to the opioid crisis, and if your kid's not ready for school, it really is not a priority for you. And they look at me when I give my parents a hard time about it. They look at me like, leave me alone; I'm doing the best I can. But it's my job to, let's go, get those babies here.

Despite pushback from parents, the principal is teaching the students how to come to school independently.

Students are doubled up (more than one family sharing a dwelling), move in and out, transient, or fall through the cracks because the school's location is in an area of prominent addiction. According to a New Hampshire school social worker:

> We have over 70 homeless students that I know of. That is over 10% of the school and we probably actually have more than that because others could be doubled up or not identified. . . . We are in an area of addiction, high poverty, and high transients. Because of all this, the students that move in and out.

In addition to homelessness, students are also removed from their homes because of addiction and temporarily live with grandparents and other caregivers, leading to a change in schools. An instructional coach explained that the frequency of moves caused by the broken foster care system and the instability of the students is tragically impacting their school day.

> We had a student held at gunpoint, and she was already in a relative foster placement. She was already removed from her biological parents'

> home because of drugs. The foster placement allowed a family member who was in jail for drugs to move back home, and a dealer held a student at gunpoint for money. Now the student cannot live with her biological parents or her relative foster placement. They are starting the process of moving the child again. There are so many of our poor little peanuts in the system moving around. They are stuck moving around in a broken system.

Multiple New Hampshire educators tell stories of students held at gunpoint and victims of serious crime as if it is just another day on the job.

On another day of conversations, the school counselor shared:

> Last year we had 300 kids in and out of this school in one year. We can have 620 kids then weeks later we have 575 kids in our school. We have a huge transient population because of drugs and homelessness. Kids can move one block and be at a different school, and they do, and we lose them, but they can come back.

The social worker added that the school works with the Family Promise Program. The Family Promise Program provides homeless families food, shelter, advocacy, and support. As described, it sounds terrific, but it adds to the transiency of the school because students could be moved to other schools through the program. The social worker explained, "We are working with the Family Promise Program, but our family is relocating all over the state every two weeks."

Transiency, poverty, and homelessness are outside environmental factors that impact attendance, learning, and consistency of services at Cobbs Hill School. The Fox Hollow United School and Anderson Loop School are experiencing similar situations.

Fox Hollow United, Maine

Similar to Cobbs Hill School, consequences of the opioid crisis, such as student transiency, homelessness, and poverty, directly impacted classrooms at Fox Hollow United. Low attendance and frequent moves were harmful to the school. According to a Maine administrator, 15% of the students who attended Fox Hollow United were homeless. The schools in the district are neighborhood schools, and various shelters are located within the city. According to the educators interviewed, students are coming and going, disappearing and reappearing, finding shelters and leaving shelters, living in foster care, moving with grandparents, and sometimes coming back and forth between schools in the district. And sometimes, students are lost and are unable to locate.

According to a Maine teacher:

> We get a lot of kids that will move and come back in two months. That happens a lot, and it's just it sucks for the kid. After leaving for a few months, they come back here, and it feels like a step back. It's hard for the teachers, we make so much progress with kids and then they just move. Eventually, they come back, and they are so much worse, and all progress is gone.

Educators expressed the difficulty of progress, regressions, and regression based on transiency. According to a social worker, "There are 301 homeless children in the district. These students are transient. The students are living in shelters, cars, camps, or outside." Students move around from city to city, from shelter to shelter, and from school to school within the district and out of the district. Sometimes they stay away, and sometimes they come back. According to a district administrator, "My guess is 40 percent of the kids that are there on the first day may not be there on the last."

The Maine principal shared the same concerns:

> We have a student whose family was dealing with addiction. She missed 43 or more days of school. We started making phone calls but never got a response. Mom was in crisis with addiction. We reached out to community police. They knocked for us. They checked in. No response. The family was moving around, unbeknownst to us. That is when we knew, we had to start an attendance team.

Later during the interview, the principal added:

> We've got an attendance team. They will buy alarm clocks for kids. They will make phone calls to kids. They will do incentives for kids, especially the older kids, because for younger kids, obviously, it's all about the parent getting the kid up and off to school. But, when they start getting into the fourth grade, some of them can do it themselves, and, unfortunately, that's probably their best chance if we give them some tools to do it themselves.

The principal explained the importance of the attendance team to track and find no-show students in an attempt to keep them attending school. Likewise, a teacher added:

> The opioid epidemic impacts my class on a lot of levels. The biggest impact is that my students are taken away. Kids are in school, then leave the school and eventually come back to school. Sometimes they are put

> in foster care or need to stay with someone else. Sometimes you have other kids suddenly missing school, and you know things are not right. You need to investigate; you need to figure it out, sometimes, it is hard to figure it out, but ultimately you will. . . . Most of the time, it takes a crisis to get to crisis point, and then the kids were taken away, and sadly we may or may not see them again.

At Fox Hollow United, educators claimed that opioid abuse leads to lost children and transient families, which directly impacts attendance, classroom, and learning. The attendance teams were created once the school felt that it was in crisis.

Similarly, Anderson Loop School is experiencing parallel challenges as Cobbs Hill and Fox Hollow.

Anderson Loop School, Massachusetts

In relation to the other two schools, Anderson Loop School teachers reported similar situations, and the impact of transiency, homelessness, poverty, and attendance were recurring themes throughout all the educator interviews. Students attending Anderson Loop School come and go throughout the school year, attending for a short time and then going missing for days or weeks. Teachers share that drug activity is a reason for many of their students' homelessness and poverty. Students move from school to school within and outside the district, from shelter to shelter. An administrator explained, "The epidemic is causing homelessness, and they stay in our school, but attendance is always affected by transportation. They have to get here. And that can often be a hardship. So, we're definitely seeing its effect in attendance." Another administrator added, "We have a huge number of homeless kids. Our children are incredibly transient; they move all around the city and back and forth between other cities. We see lots of kids in foster care because of parents' addiction."

The inconsistencies were impacting the students and the classroom. The following noteworthy quotes explain the severity of the situation at the Anderson Loop School.

According to a Massachusetts teacher:

> We have a huge number of homeless kids. Our children are incredibly transient. They move all around the city and back and forth between other cities. We see lots of kids in foster care, I have lots of cases of kids in foster care because of parents' addiction, and it's repeating the cycle. . . . I have three or four students with ten or more absences, which is a pretty big percentage of their first-grade experience. Lots of kids coming and going. I think this year, I have lost three of my students to a move, and

> I've gained two or three more who've moved into the district. I know other teachers who have lost, gained, lost, gained the same student over the school year.

An administrator added:

> We also see a lot of transients. We have families that are moving in and out of the area. We have put in a lot of time into creating services and finding the right match for teachers, and then all of a sudden, they up and move to a different part of the city, or they move to a different town or move to a different state. We know many are directly related to issues, such as incarceration, drugs, or a transition in terms of the home.

Likewise, another teacher explained:

> So, kids are transient all the time. I have had one student who already has moved three times this year, in this school year alone. She will unenrolled, which means they are no longer part of our school system. She has enrolled in another school, never goes. She never shows up to the other school and then comes back here three weeks later.

Principals, administrators, teachers, and counselors all share the same concerns over students' inconsistent attendance resulting from moves, homelessness, transiency, and foster care. Students come and go; many students eventually lost within the system; and schools feel that they do not have the tools and resources to track them or find them.

Another challenge that emerged from this theme specific to Massachusetts was that homeless students came to school from all over Massachusetts, as students and families were placed in random homeless shelters across the state. A teacher explained that she "had a student who had to travel an hour and a half drive every morning and every afternoon because the family had been placed in a shelter that was somewhere two hours away." Another teacher explained that her students had to walk to and from school because the homeless shelter was two miles away, and because schools are neighborhood schools, busing was not provided. The teacher stated, "I have had students that have been homeless, and it has been a challenge for sure. They have to walk to school two miles from the homeless shelter." She later added:

> [T]he students were, of course, late every day because they're walking two miles to and from school every day, and other students who are even further away were picked up late every day because their mother had to come and get them from the shelter across the state.

Another teacher explained that her student would show up at 12:30 because she lived so far away. The teacher said:

> Mom was struggling to get her here. Her attendance was highly affected; her academics were highly affected because she had such big gaps. She'd miss 3–4 days in a row. Or come in at 12 pm, 12:30, one o'clock when we go home at 3.

The organization and logistics of the homeless shelters seemed to be a unique challenge to Massachusetts. Educators in Maine and New Hampshire did not report transportation challenges once students were placed in homeless shelters.

Bringing It All Together

All three schools shared similar concerns regarding the challenges of constant fluctuations in student attendance. The experiences of educators emphasize common threads and viewpoints regardless of their geographical location or state. They unanimously highlighted the profound influence of transiency, homelessness, and poverty on attendance. Teachers were deeply concerned by attendance issues and their repercussions within their schools and classrooms.

Summing up the educators' perspectives, it's evident that student homelessness, transiency, poverty, neglect, household instability, and changes in guardianship had a direct bearing on attendance patterns. Teachers attributed household addiction as the underlying cause contributing to associated issues of poverty, homelessness, and transiency, leading students to shift between schools, districts, states, shelters, and caretakers. These daunting struggles and hurdles significantly impact schools, strain resources, and impede the continuity of academic and supplementary support services.

8 Bearing the Unseen Burden

Educators Struggles Amidst the Opioid Crisis in Schools

Excerpt from the Field Journal:

Yesterday, I listened to a story from, Lucina, a 20-year veteran teacher, deeply distraught over a student and an associated situation.

Lucina explained that her 20-year commitment to the community stems from being a steadfast anchor for her students, a safe haven in their lives. However, this week she found herself in an extremely difficult situation and she is still emotionally ill about how the events of that day unfolded.

Lucina's anguish stemmed from reporting a student experiencing severe abuse to the Department of Youth Services (DYS) with no response. Despite her persistent efforts, there was no callback, no visit from a DYS representative, not even an acknowledgment of the urgent situation she highlighted. Her distress amplified as it seemed her concerns weren't considered a top priority, leaving her feeling powerless and helpless, and unwilling to send the student back to a potentially harmful environment.

When the day concluded and dismissal approached, she still did not receive a call, visit, or acknowledgement from DYS, and she was instructed to release the student to go home. Fearing she'd be complicit in allowing the abuse to continue, Lucina found herself in a moment of emotional turmoil and decided to physically prevent the student from leaving and stood in front of her student's bus, not allowing the bus to depart. She understood the consequences of her actions but felt justified as her intervention finally prompted attention. The student was taken off the bus, and the administration stepped in to address the case. That night, the student didn't return home. Lucina acknowledges the extreme nature of her actions, admitting she felt like she made a better choice than her other option to "kidnap" the student and bring him home with her. Lucina does not regret her decision to stand in front of the bus and would repeat it if necessary.

Lucina's experience is just one among many documented experiences of educators in the study. It raises critical questions about how to better equip and support teachers in handling emotionally taxing and challenging circumstances.

DOI: 10.4324/9781003378204-10

The opioid crisis has posed significant challenges for school districts and students, stemming from exposure within households and environments. Consequently, schools have found themselves in crisis mode, their role extending beyond education to address issues like poor attendance and constant student turnover. Amidst this, educators have become intimately familiar with the profound trauma students face, directly impacting the emotional and physical well-being of these caring teachers. A surprising yet predominant theme emerging from interviews was the secondary trauma experienced by teachers. The needs and suffering of students profoundly affect these educators, who find themselves responsible for much more than just imparting knowledge – they become providers of basic necessities and creators of safe havens within their classrooms.

Upon analyzing the gathered data from interviews and surveys, it became clear that teachers' responsibilities have taken a nontraditional turn. The incidents witnessed have significantly affected the mental health and emotional well-being of educators, challenging their expectations in unforeseen ways. For example, in the survey, educators were asked about situations they have seen happen to students as a direct result of students' exposure to opioid exposure, and the three schools combined reported 93% (n = 62) of educators witnessed student neglect, 85% (n = 57) had a student removed from home because of an addicted family member, 76% (n = 51) witnessed student abuse, 56% (n = 37) had a student whose parent had died from opioid use, and 51% (n = 34) had students who observed an overdose. Educators also wrote about situations that their students were exposed to, such as young students being human trafficked to get parents drug money, lack of supervision, sexual abuse, homelessness, frequent moves, serious health concerns, starvation, lack of clothing and shoes, and the lack of other critical life essentials.

Teachers across all three schools acknowledged similar challenges. Through a review and analysis of survey and interview data, it became evident that teachers were notably less focused on academic achievements and more invested in ensuring students' fundamental needs were met while trying to prioritize their well-being. This emphasis led to a strong advocacy for wraparound services, aiming to cater to students' basic needs. Additionally, teachers demonstrated empathy toward students who had endured significant life traumas at such a young age. Their desire to alleviate their struggles and make life more manageable was apparent. However, these efforts left teachers feeling overwhelmed, stressed, and fatigued due to the profound impact the opioid epidemic was having on their students.

In their personal fight for consistent wraparound services, teachers went beyond their roles by purchasing clothing, jackets, and crochet hats, and even providing lunches to students in need.

A Massachusetts special education teacher shared that teachers spend so much time thinking about their students while trying to figure out ways to help:

> I know for a fact that many of the teachers on my team spend a lot of time outside of school hours worrying about their kids, thinking about their kids. I had a team of people who crocheted and knitted hats and mittens, and scarves for my students this year because we know that that's something that they need and can't always get.

In New Hampshire, a teacher shared:

> You wanna save them. I've brought in clothes, I've brought in food, I've had my kids go through their toys. I fed one girl for four months at lunch last year, given my own lunch to kids. . . . It's wearing.

Teachers also reported feeling a sense of helplessness and were overwhelmed because crises are brought to their attention. They requested help through the Department of Youth Services (referred to by educators as DYS, DCYF, or DCY), and nothing happened. Their students continued to return home to horrible situations.

For example, from September through December, a New Hampshire counselor called DYS 11 times on one family with no interventions until the 11th report, and then, the children were removed. According to the counselor:

> From September to December, we made 50 reports to DCYF. Eleven of those were just from one family. They finally got taken out of the house. We kept reporting and reporting and reporting, and it's three kids in the family.

A Maine teacher shared the same helpless feeling of frustration:

> I have to talk to DHS often about different kids and family situations, but they are so overloaded, they have told me to point blank when I've called, "I can't even think about this right now because I have to go spend a night at a hotel with a baby" so nothing happens.

As shared in the field journal, a Massachusetts teacher stood in front of a bus because she was so upset that one of her students who was being severely abused was being sent home after calling DYS.

As participants mentioned, trying to teach students within opioid epicenters was emotionally draining. Massachusetts and New Hampshire interviews revealed that multiple teachers had to take medical leave for post-traumatic stress disorder and panic attacks. A New Hampshire administrator explained:

> [L]ast year I had two very young teachers admitted to the hospital with panic attacks, never had panic attacks before in their life. There are days that I'm sure some of them just don't want to come back and try this again.

Additionally, a Massachusetts teacher explained her feelings and added that three of her colleagues had to take medical leave specifically for PTSD.

Teachers also reported parents' behaviors as "frightening and odd" and did not know how to handle various situations when encountered by a parent under the influence. Parents have verbally or physically assaulted administrators in all three locations. In combination, teachers reported that student trauma, unresponsiveness of the Department of Youth Services, parent behaviors, and unmet basic needs impacted the teacher experience, trauma, and possible retention.

What follows are specific overviews from the perspectives of teachers.

The epidemic's impact on teachers at Cobbs Hill School can be summarized and understood through the teachers' words. Throughout the interviews, teachers told stories with tears in their eyes about the impact the epidemic was having on their students. Some could not finish sentences; some changed the subject quickly when they did not want to discuss it anymore. Regardless of the added stress, fear, and anxiety, the teachers of Cobbs Hill School reported so much love and compassion for their students. According to interviews, the impact of the student's experiences impacted the teacher's well-being.

The following quotes emphasize the secondary stress and anguish the teacher experienced.

According to a special education teacher:

> I think that during the day you put on a happy face, because you know it's what the kids need to see, but then it affects you at home. Ya know, coming here and hearing about sexual abuse, and how the children have no food, and how they get food and hide it underneath . . . it's just . . . it is so wearing on everyone here, emotionally. You do become numb to it; bed bugs and lice are a daily occurrence. It's just kind of, you know, do I send a kid that has lice to the nurse every day? Because they get sent home, and I don't want that, or do I keep them where they need to be fed, warm, and safe? So, it's a constant struggle emotionally, not to . . . you know, you wanna save them. I've brought in clothes, I've brought in food, I've had my kids go through their toys. I fed one girl for four

> months at lunch last year, given my own lunch to kids, just to have them make it through the day and feel something. It's wearing. I think the trauma that . . . especially this school, the teachers and administrators feel is like nothing that I've ever seen before.

According to the principal:

> If we look at the saturation of the epidemic in the community and we see the adverse behaviors and impact on the children, my staff has clearly been affected. I mean there are this many chairs in my office because my emergency team needs time to debrief negative incidents with each other all the time. We need to meet in this office because we need each other. Last year I had two very young teachers admitted to the hospital with panic attacks; never had panic attacks before in their life. There are days that I'm sure some of them just don't want to come back and try this again. There are days that I don't want to come back and try this again. But I feel an obligation, and I think that's what they do too. We are here for our babies.

A behavior specialist added:

> I worry about my students over the weekend. Holidays, I worry about them. This is tough this role is tough. I am always worrying about them. I need to take care of myself, and sometimes I can, but most of the time, it bothers me so much that I cannot stop the worrying. In my mind, it is always them, them, them. These kids have nothing. Nothing.

A kindergarten teacher explained:

> It is so hard. I think of my babies all the time. I do not know what they are going home to after school. Are they going on to a home with a parent that overdosed that day? Will they see that? Will they be the ones to find them? Are they going home to starve and realize their parents would rather purchase drugs than feed them dinner? I don't know! Every day I wonder what my babies are going home to. They do not know what they are going home to. I do not know what they are going home to. It is so so hard.

The ramifications of the epidemic are clearly taking a toll on the teachers and their well-being. Despite all the hardships teachers encountered, the Cobbs Hill administration reported that teacher attendance is always very high because the teachers care for the children and want to be there for students.

The teachers and educators at Fox Hollow United and Anderson Loop School have similar experiences as those at Cobbs Hill School.

In an analysis of the interviews, the educators at Fox Hollow United School reported similar responses to those at Cobbs Hill School.

When the principal was asked, "How has the opioid epidemic impacted your school?", his first response was:

> The piece that probably impacts us the most about the epidemic is the impact on staff. The staff is really struggling with holding all this together. When you have that many kids in need, how do you take it in as an adult? It's hard.

Another administrator also mentioned that the teachers were "affected with their own vicarious trauma" and would love to be able to provide staff therapists. Unanticipated teacher trauma is an unanticipated consequence of the opioid epidemic.

Additionally, a teacher at the Anderson Loop School reported her anxiety when students went home for the day:

> I can't think of any teacher in my school who has not felt absolutely beaten down by all of this. We love our students, and we want what's best for our students. and it's hard to go home at the end of the day and not think about, "Are they safe? Are they getting dinner tonight? What adult is with them right now? Will I see them again tomorrow?"

Teachers at Anderson Loop School explained that they are stressed, exhausted, and feel a sense of helplessness. They do not feel as if they have the proper training to address the needs of the students exposed to the opioid epidemic.

A first-grade teacher explained that a student watched her mom's murder. The teacher reached out for help to the central office administration. She was hoping for support for herself and the student, but instead, they gave her a pamphlet to read, and that was the only support she was offered. Another teacher explained that in her short tenure at Anderson Loop School, "three teachers had to take medical leave for PTSD."

Another teacher added:

> It's exhausting. It is absolutely and completely exhausting. I mean, I'm young. I'm only 26, and I come home from work just exhausted. I go to bed at eight o'clock because I just feel so fried from trying to understand what my kids are going through, how to figure out how to help them. That is the emotional part of it, of just, "Oh, my gosh. They're sitting here crying. They're not crying over my math lesson; there's something else in the picture." I so badly want to be the constant for them, the support for them, but obviously, I need to be taking care of myself a bit more in that process, too.

The collection of teacher's stories, words, and experiences expressed robust evidence of the anguish, confusion, and worry teachers experience daily in opioid-crisis regions. The prevailing words of the educators indicate that their students' experiences and traumas directly influence their well-being.

Bringing It All Together

Educators at all three schools reported similar stories and concerns. Teachers say that they are exhausted and need more support in helping the challenging situations they are exposed to. The needs, neglect, and pain of students are impacting teachers. Teachers are responsible for more than just educating students. Teachers provide students with basic needs they do not receive at home and create a safe haven in their classrooms. The exposed secondary trauma of educators was an unexpected theme that emerged within the study and is worthy of more in-depth investigation in the future.

Educators from all three schools shared parallel narratives and expressed shared concerns. They conveyed their exhaustion and emphasized the need for increased support in managing the demands of the challenging student population they serve. The evident needs, neglect, and distress experienced by students significantly affect the educator's well-being. Way beyond their primary role of imparting knowledge, teachers are assuming the responsibility of addressing students' unmet basic needs and fostering a secure environment, creating safe havens within their classrooms.

One notable and unforeseen aspect revealed in the study was the secondary trauma experienced by educators – an area that warrants further comprehensive exploration in future investigations.

9 Navigating the Challenges

School Preparedness and Special Education

Excerpt from the Field Journal:

During the interview process, I would ask numerous questions about academic achievement, and many times, that question was glossed over, leading down a different, participant-led conversation path.

The interviewee's reaction to my academic focus questions made me think about my first-hand experiences in the schools and how the academic responsibility of teachers may be far less important than the responsibilities of keeping their students safe, fed, warm, clean, and cared for.

I started this research to understand the changes in special education and the academic impact of schools in opioid-crisis regions. Within the first few weeks, I was overwhelmed with the overall experiences of everyone involved. I quickly began to see that it seemed as if educators were asking for help and sharing stories, hoping that public awareness would lead to the resources they need to care for their students. Many times during the interviews, my questions were answered, but the conversations continued to evolve in a purposeful participant-led direction. Notably, the direction of the conversation was remarkably similar in all the interviews, regardless of school, titles, and geographic location.

We were experiencing a crisis – men, women, and children across the country are suffering, and many times, by no fault of their own, but rather the results of the severe ramifications of a public health emergency. This public health crisis is no longer dormant in schools- it is in the open, and the burden is felt by educators, students, and the surrounding community.

Throughout this investigation, it was notable how insignificant educators seemed to perceive the topic of academic achievement. Not that this is an unimportant area to investigate, but in conversations, it seemed irrelevant compared to the day-to-day challenge's educators experienced. Initially, the project aimed to uncover shifts and impacts on special education and

DOI: 10.4324/9781003378204-11

academic progress. However, a few weeks in, it became clear that educators did not view this as their primary concern. Their focus leaned more toward the survival and well-being of their students, with a far less significant emphasis on academic achievements. Chapter 9 delves into evidence from special education documents, district statistics, curriculum assessments, surveys, and interviews. It aims to create a comprehensive overview of how the opioid crisis affects resources, interventions, special education, how educators perceive their readiness to support students affected by this epidemic, and what solutions and measures districts are implementing.

As highlighted by participants and detailed in earlier chapters, external factors significantly affect students. The lives these students lead and their experiences beyond school – exposure to drugs, crime, neglect, and unstable parental/guardian situations – directly influence their academic performance. Educators also noted that students arrive at school anxious, lacking motivation, easily distracted, and displaying evident signs of trauma and emotional challenges. Consequently, there's a prioritization of mental health support and basic life necessities over academic pursuits. Are educators in regions affected by the opioid crisis adequately trained to meet the needs of these exposed children? Are schools equipped for these challenges? Are schools prepared?

Special Education

According to data collected from internal documents and publicly available statistics, the percentage of students who receive special education services has remained the same within the few years this initial study took place (2017–2019). All three schools stayed within the same approximate percentages of students identified as having a disability and receiving special education services from 2017 to 2019. Teachers and principals perceived the number was increasing, but according to publicly available data from each state education department, those numbers remained relatively the same within those years. However, it is noteworthy that in 2019, all three school districts mentioned that their kindergarten special education numbers were the highest they had ever seen (in Chapter 12, there is a 2023 follow-up investigation to see if those predictions are solidified). It is also remarkable that, according to district administrations, two out of the three schools increased interventions before students qualified to receive special education services. Increasing interventions was a district-wide initiative to keep the special education numbers from increasing. According to the administration, increasing interventions and remediations were the school's attempt to minimize special education services by providing increased services before the special education referral process.

According to a Massachusetts administrator, "Students need probably a minimum of 20 interventions at least be exhausted, then we would start to think about the possibility of SPED." In addition, a Maine administrator noted:

> While I don't see our SPED number going up, referrals for support are going way up, but the level of supports that we've had to put in place to keep them in the classroom without special education services and keeping kids in the least restrictive environment has gone way up.

Furthermore, all three schools mentioned that students coming into kindergarten with identified disabilities had increased dramatically this year. According to a Massachusetts special education teacher, "Caseloads seem to be getting larger and larger. I know in our incoming kindergarten class this year, we have 18 already on IEPs. That is a crazy number for kindergarten to come in with." Both Maine and New Hampshire participants indicated the same situation with students coming from preschool:

According to the New Hampshire principal:

> I just met with my SPED team this morning, we have 28 kindergartners coming in in the fall that are identified with special needs. Twenty-eight coming from the child find! I need another kindergarten teacher and another special education teacher because that is an entire caseload of students right there.

According to a district administrator in Maine:

> I just heard in a meeting that we're inheriting kids with more needs than ever before, kids are showing up for kindergarten with greater needs than ever before. And I'm sure, my assumption is that it is linked to this epidemic.

All three schools are impacted by the number of kindergarteners or incoming kindergarteners who need special education services. The plethora of needs identified in children exposed to the epidemic – whether receiving special education or not – could make one wonder if the teachers were prepared to teach and address the needs of the students. The following section examines the educator's perceived preparation to support students with diverse needs.

Knowledge and Preparation for Opioid Exposure and Disabilities

As highlighted in Chapter 2 and according to the literature and published research, children with Neonatal Abstinence Syndrome (NAS) who were exposed to opioids in utero could have a cognitive or language deficit (Beckwith & Burke, 2015; Fill et al., 2018; Kim et al., 2021; McGlone & Mactier, 2015; Nygaard et al., 2015; Ornoy et al., 2010; Yuan et al., 2014). The possibility of such disabilities could qualify children for special education services for academic challenges. Additionally, evidence suggests that students who are living in the care of a parent or household with someone struggling with an opioid-use disorder may be at higher risk of experiencing trauma, school absences, social withdrawal, and behavior issues that can contribute to impacting educational outcomes (Crouch, 2019; Drescher et al., 2022; Herranz et al., 2014; Jimenez et al., 2016; Nunes et al., 2015; Peisch et al., 2018). Such experiences and challenges could lead to a disability diagnosis and could possibly qualify students for special education services. In addition to the direct link between parents and children, community drug use and exposure in the child's expanded social environment and network outside the home is also linked to negative consequences for the development of children (Wolf et al., 2016). These possible outcomes of the opioid epidemic impact the children's ability to learn, engage, and thrive in school.

As stated above, a child exposed to the opioid epidemic could have experienced trauma and adverse childhood experiences (ACEs) leading to behavioral, cognitive, social, and emotional disabilities. During the case-study investigation, the percentage of educators trained to tackle the associated disabilities was revealed through survey results, interviews, and an analysis of internal professional development offerings. Since two of the three districts are increasing interventions prior to special education referrals, the general education teacher will be responsible for addressing the needs of the students unless the students receive special education services. Therefore, the knowledge of and training for associated disabilities should be universal to maximize benefits for all educators.

According to survey results, in the combined three case studies (MA, ME, and NH), 83% (n = 56) of educators have training in trauma, 73% (n = 48) in social-emotional disabilities, and 71% (n = 47) feel the most prepared to teach students with ADHD. According to educators, mental illness is another symptom of their student's exposure to opioid abuse or the ramifications of the opioid crisis. Unfortunately, only 25% (n = 16) of participating educators have been trained in mental disorders and illness, and only 33% (n = 22) feel prepared to teach someone with a mental disorder. Notably, only 8% (n = 5) of educators received training or professional development specific to the opioid epidemic and NAS, and only 21% (n = 14) of participating educators feel prepared to teach a student who was born with NAS or has been exposed to opioid use.

Teachers are not the only ones with concerns about preparation. During an interview with the New Hampshire principal, questions were asked regarding resources. The interview took place in January 2019. During the interview, she explained her perceived understanding of the district's response to the crisis. She explained that she had raised her concerns about the opioid epidemic and the impact on schools in 2016 when she supervised Child Find. Child Find is part of the Individuals with Disabilities Education Act (IDEA), and under federal law, public schools must look for, find, and evaluate kids who possibly need special education. Three years prior to our conversation, the principal recalled that over 400 students were evaluated for a possible disability and in need of special education services because of maternal substance overuse during pregnancy. She reached out to district administration about her concerns over these numbers and the root cause of the increase in evaluations, but, according to her, the expressed concerns were ignored. According to the principal:

> Districts and schools are woefully unprepared. We are woefully unprepared. When I supervised child find before I was the principal here, in one year three years ago, we brought in more than 400 preschoolers for evaluation. Most of those young children were evaluated because there was a substance abuse issue when mom was pregnant. We knew that three years ago. Three years ago! We have not prepared for those children in our district. We know, but we are not addressing the needs of those children in our schools, and we are still not preparing for them. It is like if we ignore it, maybe it will go away or get better . . . nope! My concerns were shared three years ago. Nothing has been done. We have not prepared ourselves for the surge of students impacted by the opioid epidemic. Our response is terrible, but I do not think you will find a place prepared for this. How can you prepare for this? We are all just running on a shoestring.

Administration and teachers seem to agree in all three school districts, and the analysis of three years of professional development documents (2016 through 2019) proves that the school districts have not proactively focused on preparing teachers for the social-emotional and academic needs of students impacted by the communities in crisis.

During interviews, several teachers mentioned that they have students in their classes who were notified of being born with NAS. However, requests to the district for further details, suggested accommodations, and expected behaviors were not provided. Teachers were left investigating and learning on their own as described by a special education teacher in Maine.

> NAS has affected my students. I have students who were born addicted to opiates. And the biggest problem is there's no research on it. So, there's nothing out there yet about how that affects the brain and how that affects development. There's a ton about Fetal Alcohol Syndrome, but

> nothing about being born addicted to opiates. The one student that I do have this year, that we know was born addicted to opiates, was adopted. And it's hard for that parent to find solutions and find resources because we don't know, they don't know, I don't know, and there's no research out there.

That interview revealed that this teacher is knowledgeable about NAS, seeking resources and researching the effects, but is unsuccessful in finding literature to help her in the classroom.

During 13 of the 29 interviews, teachers from the three schools who worked with students with NAS described some of the challenges. When reviewing the 13 educators who mentioned NAS, they stated that students with NAS have been observed having aggressive behaviors, socially inappropriate reactions, academic delays, emotional regulation issues, inability to de-escalate, explosive reactions, and anxiety. These were the educators' observations and perceptions shared during the interviews, but further research is needed in this area. It cannot be proved that these behaviors described by the educators are the consequence of NAS or other competing reasons. This is noteworthy, however, because of the consistency of behaviors described by multiple educators in this study.

Overall Perceived Preparedness

Teachers expressed concerns that they were not equipped or trained to address the needs of their students exposed to the ramifications and impact of the opioid crisis in the classroom. The administration also had concerns regarding overall preparedness and external/internal resources to address the needs of the school, students, and staff. Overall, 100% ($N = 29$) of the interview participants in all three case studies and locations felt unprepared.

When asked about support to address the needs of students affected by the opioid crisis, most expressed words of helplessness. For example, a situation shared by a first-grade teacher describes her helplessness. The teacher did not know what to do or how to respond when a first-grade student, playing with Barbies, reenacts a drug bust and pretends to flush drugs down the toilet. Another teacher does not know what to do when students talk about their parents' deaths.

> Last year, I had a mother who was killed in front of my student, so I specifically asked the central office for support, and I was handed a packet to read, and that was it. It came from downtown, and that was the most we got. That was after reaching out, specifically reaching out for help about this. I did not know what to do!

The teacher explained that she had to seek help from a doctor on her own because she wanted to make sure it was addressed correctly.

Here are a few notable expressions of concern when interview participants were asked, "What is your district/school doing to proactively prepare for the influx of students impacted by the epidemic, either born with NAS or living in an environment exposed to the opioid epidemic?"

- We are not having professional development on the crisis. As teachers, we have not been trained in anything related to the opioid epidemic. We need to know. We need to understand. I do not know what to do about it. We have not learned anything about it (New Hampshire P3, Personal Communication, February 2019).
- The teachers are not equipped to deal with the amount of trauma sitting in front of them, and they're not supported enough to deal with that. And it's a hard job. It's a hard job in our district because accountability is so high. In a district like this, we are under the microscope all the time. And it's extremely difficult to teach when you have children that are struggling with trauma. Because to those children school does not matter. The trauma that they're dealing with is so much bigger than learning and passing the MCAS. They could care less about school because their world is so shattered. . . . But state concern is that we need to increase those MCAS scores (Massachusetts P7, Personal Communication, January 2019).
- We're just not trained for this. When you go to school to be a teacher, no one teaches you how to deal with any of these behaviors, all of the absences, the tardiness, things like that, or how to deal with like my student this year whose mother passed away, talks about it all the time. I don't know how to handle that, as a classroom teacher. What do I say to him? Do I let him talk about it but not in front of the other kids? Then the other kids, he'll talk about it at recess. How do I handle it with them? It's definitely straining and dealing with the behaviors is exhausting (Massachusetts P4, Personal Communication, January 2018).
- Unfortunately, I don't think a lot. They could probably be doing more. But, no I wouldn't say there's been any opportunities to learn more or prepare (New Hampshire P7, Personal Communication, January 2019).
- I think that we fall really short in that regard. It's been acknowledged, the need for more professional development and support has been acknowledged. But it's not there yet. (Massachusetts P2, Personal Communication, January 2019).
- I would say nothing. I think they know it's a problem, I just think it's . . . in this district itself, it's really overwhelming, where we don't know where to start (New Hampshire P6, Personal Communication, January 2019).
- I do not feel like my school district has done anything for me at this point in time. I mean, I'm a fairly young teacher. I had my training fairly recently.

I have not had any trauma training or anything specific to the opioid crisis (Massachusetts P6, Personal Communication, January 2019).

- I could be wrong, but I don't think the district is doing anything to prepare us. I don't feel very supported, or I don't know that there's much proactivity going on. We all know about it. We talk about it. But nothing is getting done (Massachusetts P5, Personal Communication, January 2019).
- I don't think we're doing very much that I'm aware of. I mean, we've discussed it a little bit here in this building throughout our principal and administration, and I've had private conversations with them when things have happened in the room. But I don't think we are doing anything that I'm aware of (Massachusetts P3, Personal Communication, January 2019).
- I guess I don't know. I'm not sure, I have not been involved in any specific training through the school district around that (New Hampshire P8, Personal Communication, January 2019).
- As teachers, we haven't been trained. It is so hard. I don't know what to do with the whole situation. We just haven't learned anything about it (New Hampshire P3, Personal Communication, February 2019).
- We are woefully unprepared (New Hampshire P1, Personal Communication, January 2019).

According to 100% of interview participants ($N = 29$), districts are falling short of acknowledging the challenges and supporting those working with students impacted by this national crisis. However, further investigation shows that the districts have attempted some solutions that teachers may or may not be aware of. Chapter 10 will dive into professional development plans, administrative interviews, and district documents to share attempted initiatives uncovered that school-based educators may not have been aware of or exposed to.

Bringing It All Together

Educators prioritized addressing the nonacademic needs of students over academics in opioid epidemic crisis regions. While academics were not disregarded, educators allocated most of their interview time to discussing basic student needs.

Across three districts, despite a rise in intervention referrals, special education services remained consistent between 2017 and 2019. There is a prediction that those numbers will rise with the incoming Kindergarten class for the 2019–2020 school year based on preschool interventions and initial numbers (Chapter 12 will revisit this prediction). However, teachers expressed feeling ill-equipped to support students affected by the opioid crisis, with 100% of participants stating their districts are not proactively preparing for the influx of students impacted by the opioid epidemic entering their schools. The districts lacked acknowledgment, adequate professional development, and support for these students. Surveys indicated that only 21% of educators felt ready to teach affected students, with a mere 8% reporting any relevant training.

References

Beckwith, A. M., & Burke, S. A. (2015). Identification of early developmental deficits in infants with prenatal heroin, methadone, and other opioid exposure. *Clinical Pediatrics, 54*(4), 328. https://doi.org/10.1177/0009922814549545

Crouch, E., Radcliff, E., Hung, P., & Bennett, K. (2019). Challenges to school success and the role of adverse childhood experiences. *Academic Pediatrics, 19*(8), 899–907. https://doi-org.proxy3.noblenet.org/10.1016/j.acap.2019.08.006

Drescher, J., Steyer, L., Townley-Flores, C., & Humphreys, K. (2022). Has the opioid crisis affected student learning? A national analysis of growth rates. *The ANNALS of the American Academy of Political and Social Science, 703*(1), 234–261. https://doi.org/10.1177/00027162231151524

Fill, M. A., Miller, A. M., Wilkinson, R. H., Warren, M. D., Dunn, J. R., Schaffner, W., & Jones, T. F. (2018). Educational disabilities among children born with neonatal abstinence syndrome. *Pediatrics, 142*(3). https://doi.org/10.1542/peds.2018-0562

Herranz, G. S., Vílchez, M. A. L., Ledo, J. D., & Sierra, A. M. (2014). Children born to heroin-addicted mothers: What's the outcome 25 years later? *Journal of Addiction Research and Therapy, 5*(180). https://www.omicsonline.org/open-access/children-born-to-heroinaddicted-mothers-whats-the-outcome-years-later-2155-6105-1000180.php?aid=25615

Jimenez, M. E., Wade, R., Lin, Y., Morrow, L. M., & Reichman, N. E. (2016). Adverse experiences in early childhood and kindergarten outcomes. *Pediatrics, 137*(2), 2015–1839.

Kim, H. M., Bone, R. M., McNeill, B., Lee, S. J., Gillon, G., & Woodward, L. J. (2021). Preschool language development of children born to women with an opioid use disorder. *Children, 8*(4), 268. https://doi.org/10.3390/children8040268.

McGlone, L., & Mactier, H. (2015). Infants of opioid-dependent mothers: Neurodevelopment at six months. *Early Human Development, 91*(1), 19–21.

Nunes, E., Weissman, M., Goldsten, R., McAvay, G., Beckford, C., Seracini, A., & Wickramaratne, P. (2015). Psychiatric disorders and impairment in the children of opiate addicts: Prevalence and distribution by ethnicity. *American Journal on Addictions, 9*(3), 232–241.

Nygaard, E., Moe, V., Slinning, K., & Walhoyd, K. (2015). Longitudinal cognitive development of children born to mothers with opioid and polysubstance use. *Pediatric Research, 78*(3), 330–335.

Ornoy, A., Daka, L., Goldzweig, G., Gil, Y., Mjen, L., Levit, S., Shufman, E., Bar-Hamburger, R., & Greenbaum, C. (2010). Neurodevelopmental and psychological assessment of adolescents born to drug-addicted parents: Effects of SES and adoption. *Child Abuse & Neglect, 34*(5), 354–368.

Peisch, V., Sullivan, A. D., Breslend, N. L., Benoit, R., Sigmon, S. C., Forehand, G. L., Strolin-Goltzman, J., & Forehand, R. (2018). Parental opioid abuse:

A review of child outcomes, parenting, and parenting interventions. *Journal of Child and Family Studies*, *27*(7), 2082–2099. https://doi.org/10.1007/s10826-018-1061-0

Wolf, P., Ponicki, W., Kepple, N. J., & Gaidus, A. (2016, September). Are community-level prescription opioid overdoses associated with child harm? A spatial analysis of California zip codes, 2001–2011. *Drug and Alcohol Dependence*, *166*, 202–208. https://doi.org/10.1016/j.drugalcdep.2016.07.014.

Yuan, Q., Rubic, M., Seah, J., Rae, C., Wright, I. M., Kaltenbach, K., Feller, J. M., Abdel-Latif, M. E., Chu, C., & Oei, J. L. (2014). Do maternal opioids reduce neonatal regional brain volumes? A pilot study. *Journal of Perinatology*, *34*(12), 909–913. https://doi.org/10.1038/jp.2014.111

10 Unveiling Layers of Support and Need of Schools Located in Opioid Crisis Regions

Thoughts from the Field Journal:

> Today is a good day. After months of listening to serious concerns and heart-breaking stories, I met with a mental health clinician in Maine who works at the central office. The conversation was full of hope. He is newly hired and is charged with improving the student's mental health. He has goals to hire mental health clinicians in each school, create universal programs to address trauma in schools, and create a multi-tiered support program involving teachers, nurses, mental health providers, and community representatives to address the needs of the students. Although in its infancy, the plan sounds promising and innovative.

Participating educators unanimously agreed that their school districts were ill-equipped to handle the consequences of the opioid epidemic within their communities and schools. Only 21% felt adequately prepared to assist students grappling with challenges ranging from trauma and mental health disorders to community implications and potential cognitive and social-emotional disabilities resulting from the epidemic's impact on children. Shockingly, 100% of interview participants ($N = 29$) expressed a lack of proactive measures in their schools to brace for an increase in affected students. Just 8% of respondents ($n = 5$) reported feeling adequately equipped to support children affected by the opioid crisis, according to survey data.

Further examination of curriculum materials, interviews with district-level administrators, and thematic coding revealed some documented efforts – both successful and unsuccessful – to address certain needs arising from the opioid epidemic within these districts.

While these solutions weren't specifically tailored to aid children impacted by the epidemic, the case-study investigations uncovered various initiatives implemented by schools to support the broader student body, inadvertently benefiting those affected by the crisis. Each school in different states adopted unique approaches and solutions. Common measures across all

DOI: 10.4324/9781003378204-12

three institutions included providing medical and dental assessments and care when needed, supplying free food and weather-appropriate clothing, and offering before- and after-school programs to ensure a safe environment outside regular school hours.

This chapter will share some district-specific solutions and the overall needs discussed by schools located in crisis regions.

Attempted Solutions

There were some solutions in place for schools in opioid crisis areas; however, educators may not have been aware of them due to a disconnect between educators' perceptions and the available assistance, or the interventions were not shared throughout the districts. According to the analysis of school documents, professional development plans, and interviews with district-level administrators, schools did have some effective practices and interventions that addressed the educator's mentioned needs of students. The activities and assistance that support the needs of educators and students specifically address the following research question: How are schools located in opioid-crisis regions proactively preparing for the influx of students affected by the opioid epidemic entering the school? Based on the findings of this study, schools were not proactively preparing. In fact, they were reactive in addressing these needs. Still, some solutions were unintentionally in place that addressed the needs of schools regarding the influx of students affected by the opioid epidemic.

Although not directly credited as support for the needs of children impacted by the opioid epidemic, Fox Hollow School in Maine added some helpful support for students in need, such as a district-wide focus on mental health and equity. This focus included adding mental health service providers in schools and attempts to provide social-emotional learning.

At Fox Hollow, a mental health administrator was hired to oversee and support the district's school-based social workers and mental health providers. The position of director of clinical and behavior supports was located at the central office directly under the assistant superintendent of teaching and learning and was a newly developed academic position. The director currently in the position holds a Ph.D. in clinical psychology and has experience in day treatment facilities, mental health clinical supervision, experience with the implementation of social-emotional learning (SEL), and trauma-sensitive practices. As noted in multiple interviews and other documents, the director of clinical and behavior supports is credited for reviewing the district's schools' trauma-informed practices and SEL initiatives. The director was interviewed and explained his role in the system, specifically at the school level. He said that the SEL initiative was part of a multi-tiered intervention process, and he specifically guides the interventions for social/emotional and behavioral needs, working collaboratively with the school's social workers, social-emotional learning coach, and administration.

Fox Hollow also had an SEL coach who worked with the director of clinical and behavioral support and collaborated with the social workers. The responsibility of the SEL coach was to ensure adequate tier-one social-emotional supports and focus on positive behavior intervention and support.

Additionally, Fox Hollow had a before-school breakfast program that is part of the tier-one social-emotional support initiative. Before school, students were given an opportunity to check in with school social workers, administration, the SEL coach, and teachers to make sure they were ready to learn and if anything needed to be discussed that may hinder learning for the day.

Fox Hollow also had social workers with specific roles who assisted students. Some school-based social workers supported student's mental health needs, and a McKinney-Vento social worker served homeless students. The McKinney-Vento Homeless Assistance Act protects homeless students. At the time of this study, the Maine district had a substantial homeless population, so the school had a specific social worker to protect the homeless student's rights, develop a relationship with the homeless families, keep data on homeless numbers, make sure transportation was provided for families regardless of location, and track homeless students who were not showing up at school. According to the McKinney-Vento social worker, her job was to "help the most invisible, the most vulnerable population in a very concrete but powerful way, so that I can hold them and help them, get them the next step of services they need, and to properly account for them." At the time of the research in 2019, there were over 300 homeless students in the school district. Many of the homeless were a result of generational poverty or were from refugee families and drug-addicted families. The McKinney-Vento social worker is also part of the multi-tiered referral clinical team that ensures all students are receiving mental health and behavioral support and interventions before the special education referral process.

In addition to the director of clinical and behavioral support, the school district had an equity director. The equity director is a district-wide administrator position that falls under the assistant superintendent. The equity director's goal is to put systems in place to close the gap in achievement between students in the district. The equity director runs systems to ensure that schools focus on achievement, teaching the whole student, equity, and providing opportunities to focus on the people and families within the community. The overall initiative led by the equity director serves as an essential blueprint to guide student learning. In the interview process, it was evident that teachers, social workers, and administrators knew the importance of teaching the whole child and bridging the gap between school and community.

The equity director explained that a lot of time is devoted to looking at the whole child and the importance of documenting changes in behavior, academic achievement, and physical appearance, and if changes happen, the focus is on why and what is happening at home. The equity director then schedules home visits and investigates the situation.

Similar to Fox Hollow, Anderson Loop School in Massachusetts had support in place to address some of the school's needs. The school had programs to ensure that their students had opportunities for before- and after-school programs, free breakfast and free lunch, a truant/attendance officer, family resource center, and counselors were available.

The truant/attendance officer was a district-wide position with a focus on eliminating chronic absenteeism. The officer visited homes, made calls, and emailed with the goal of locating students who did not show up for school for an extended period. The truant officer located missing students and brought them to "district student court," and the court decided if the reason for extended absences was excusable. The officer's role was to eliminate the likelihood of lost children. The school attempted to keep track of absences by having this officer available. Fox Hollow School in Maine had a similar attendance solution system in place, but instead of one truant/attendance officer for the entire district, the Maine district had attendance teams at each of their schools with the same goal – to recover students who were not in school, find out why they were absent, and support them as they return.

Finally, Cobbs Hill School in New Hampshire was working to address the needs of children impacted by trauma and the opioid epidemic through a number of programs. Cobbs Hill focused on providing its students with clothing, food, warmth, safety, dental and medical services, and a variety of programs that focused on resilience, trauma-informed instruction, and mental health needs.

Cobbs Hill School received a grant to provide mental health services to students at the school during school hours. The service provider was located on-site and met and worked with students and families throughout the day. This was a city-wide initiative to improve mental health. During this study, there was an opportunity to spend the day with and interview the mental health provider to learn more about the position and role. She explained that the grant's goal and her presence in the school was to help improve the health indicators in the city. She worked with students who are living in families where there is active drug use, families who are struggling with homelessness due to past use, and children living with extended family members, whether that's an aunt or a grandparent, because of parental drug use and parent incarceration. During several interviews, other participants credited her presence as extremely valuable.

In addition to mental health support, Cobbs Hill School used a resilience curriculum. Throughout the school, there was a "Toolbox 12 Tool Poster" in every classroom, hallway, cafeteria, bathroom, and office. The poster, Visual 10.1, outlines 12 tools that can be used to help students build resilience, self-mastery, and empathy. The language of the Toolbox Project Program is used throughout the building, and the frequent use of the tools was evident when talking to interview participants. The goal was to provide tools to reinforce resilience for students who may need them and provide a visual reference throughout the day. Interview participants credited the Dovetail Project (n.d.) and the Toolbox Project Program (n.d.) as a successful calming process to avoid a crisis in the school. The poster shown in Visual 10.1 lists tools for learning and tools for life.

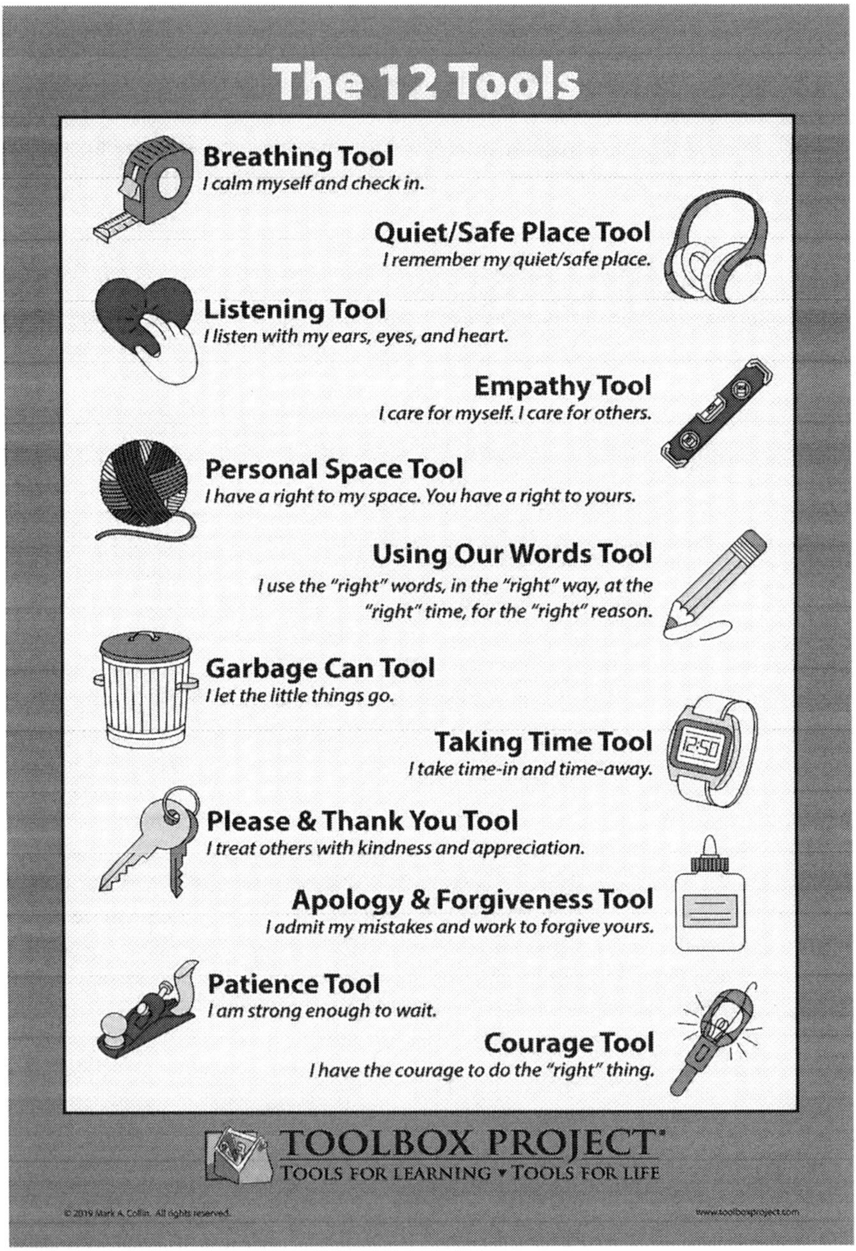

Figure 10.1 The toolbox

When students are overwhelmed, challenged, angry, sad, or frustrated, staff points to the posted "Toolbox" so that students can decide on how to react using the suggested "tools." Depending on the situation, the student will use an appropriate tool to address the issue or feeling they are experiencing.

In addition to providing mental health services, the Dovetail Project, and the Toolbox Program, a trauma consultant was hired at Cobbs Hill School to provide professional development on the benefits of creating a trauma-sensitive school. The trauma consultant was interviewed to better understand her vision. She explained that her role was to teach educators how to intervene and help students understand how their experiences contribute to their behavior, cognition, and emotions and share tools and resources on how educators can help students build security, safety, and hope moving forward. There is a specific language used with the trauma-responsive framework and practice exercises. The professional development goal is to foster reflective thinking, especially in the presence of strong emotions, to help heal students in traumatizing circumstances. The professional development also addressed dysregulated educators and maintaining composure in the face of dysregulated students. The trauma-sensitive training aimed to inform educators and provide background understanding and trauma-informed strategies to move forward.

During the investigation, the trauma program was in its infancy stage and not yet implemented, but it was an upcoming initiative that would continue for two years. This program was another grant-funded program unique to Cobbs Hill School – no other school in the district would implement the program.

All three schools provide their students with some needed basic necessities. The basic needs are met first and foremost before learning can begin by providing students with food, clothing, boots, jackets, lunch, breakfast, dental needs, medical check-ins, warmth, and safety. Additionally, at the Cobbs Hill School in New Hampshire, over 100 students go home on Friday with backpacks full of food so they can make it through the weekend until school starts again on Monday.

As noted above, some supports should be highlighted in the district's attempt to help the neediest of children. Each school has its own supports in place. Although not credited with supporting the children of the opioid epidemic, the following initiatives, revealed by interview participants, observations, survey data, and collected district-wide documents, support some of the children in need who are impacted by the epidemic.

- social workers;
- McKinney-Vento social worker;
- director of clinical and behavior supports;
- equity director;
- resilience programs;

- multi-tiered support system – social, emotional, and behavioral supports;
- professional development on poverty, trauma, resilience, and social-emotional learning;
- before- and after-school programs that provide meals and a safe place;
- mental health providers at the school.

Focusing on basic needs and the whole child – providing dental, medical, and eye care at school, free meals and snacks, free weather-appropriate clothing, and a safe place to stay.

Schools' Additional Needs

As one might imagine, the needs expressed per school for all three case studies are plentiful. The needs were based on the participants' interviews, the survey, and document collection and analysis. Generally speaking, many of the needs overlapped in each district. All three districts identified staffing as a concern, especially with the need to provide extra interventions for all students with social-emotional, behavioral, and trauma impacts. Participants acknowledged that special education caseloads are very high and could benefit from additional teachers. Furthermore, the need for more paraprofessional help was mentioned numerous times during the interviews in all three locations. In addition to staffing, participants felt they needed to learn more about Neonatal Abstinence Syndrome (NAS) and all disabilities associated with the epidemic. Parent behaviors were also a concern, and educators wanted to know how to handle and navigate parental behaviors to develop and establish better relationships. Unquestionably, budget and funding were a primary concern, especially since all district needs are dependent on appropriate funding to execute.

Based on in-depth conversations with administrators, teachers, and counselors in conjunction with reviews of curriculum and professional development plans, the following resources would be beneficial for addressing the needs of the students and educators affected by the opioid crisis (Welby, 2019). Here is a brief overview and will be revisited in greater depth in Chapter 14:

- additional special educators, behavior intervention specialists, support staff, and paraprofessionals;
- full-time mental health providers located in the schools available all day for student support, as well as interdisciplinary clinical intervention teams of mental health providers, nurses, and social workers who work together and support students and families;
- social workers who specialize in homeless populations;
- additional truancy/attendance officers in every school to keep track of students' whereabouts and no-shows;

- a district-wide resilience and social-emotional curriculum;
- professional development on the opioid crisis, particularly NAS and possible disabilities associated with opioid exposure;
- professional development on adverse childhood experiences, trauma-informed schools, trauma-sensitive teaching, and supporting students with mental health needs;
- greater support for teachers and school staff, including resilience training, professionally guided group therapy, conflict resolution, and wellness trainers for educators.

Other district needs include:

- money to sustain and expand mental health programs in school;
- increased community programs and resources that can be utilized in schools;
- training on relationship building with parents;
- more administrative training on social-emotional learning and trauma-informed practices;
- a better system or protocol between the school and the Department of Youth Services;
- solutions for transiency between schools in the same district, district-wide consistencies for policy;
- more solutions for the homeless population of students and better transportation opportunities.

The above needs were shared and uncovered in document reviews and during interviews and surveys. These needs will be revisited in Chapter 14. Based on the educator's perceptions, these needs were perceived as areas of improvement to combat the impacts and ramifications of the opioid epidemic in schools in crisis areas. Such improvements would involve increased funding and additional staff.

Bringing It All Together

Research into curriculum documents, professional development plans, discussions with district-level officials, and thematic analysis reveal a range of documented efforts, some successful while others less so, aimed at tackling the challenges linked to the opioid crisis within districts.

While not all solutions directly targeted the children impacted by the opioid epidemic, case studies demonstrated that schools adopted multiple programs benefiting the broader student body, consequently aiding affected children. Across various states, each school took different approaches.

Common initiatives encompass medical and dental checkups, providing clothing, free meals, and both pre- and after-school activities.

Moreover, extensive discussions with administrators, educators, and counselors, coupled with reviews of documents, highlighted the necessity for additional resources to support students and educators affected by the opioid crisis. Unfortunately, many of these needs hinge on increased funding and a suitable budget for implementing and sustaining such initiatives.

References

Dovetail Project. (n.d.). *Better fathers. Brighter futures.* https://thedovetailproject.org/

The ToolBox Project. (n.d). *Tools for learning. Tools for life.* https://toolboxproject.com/

Welby, K. A. (2019). Coping with the opioid crisis: Teachers need support, right now. *Phi Delta Kappan*, *101*(3), 53–56.

Part 3

Extended Research, Discussion, and Interventions

The chapters in Part 3 reveal the complex interplay between the opioid epidemic, students, teachers, schools, district leadership, and society. Part 3, which includes Chapters 11–14, consolidates and calibrates all findings from the three sites and includes two post-pandemic research studies, one as a follow-up with the original case-study participants and the other to prove external validity. The discussion explores the connections to theories, literature, and current national education trends. By linking findings to national issues such as teacher attrition, chronic absenteeism, and the broader teacher shortage crisis, the study positions its findings within the larger educational landscape. Equally important is how the research findings highlighted in Part 3 contribute to practical interventions and solutions for further investigations and offer actionable steps to address the challenges identified. Part 3 highlights the potential to inform education policies and practices, especially in regions impacted by the opioid epidemic.

DOI: 10.4324/9781003378204-13

11 Schools in Opioid-Crisis Regions

Key Findings

> We had a student held at gunpoint, and she was already in a relative foster placement. She was removed from her biological parents' home because of drugs. The foster parents allowed a family member who was in jail for drugs to move back home and a dealer broke in and held my student at gunpoint for money. Now the student cannot live with her biological parents or her relative foster placement. They are starting the process of moving the child again. There are so many of our poor little peanuts in the system just moving around. They are stuck moving around in a broken system.
>
> – Matilda, New Hampshire Instructional Coach

In the prior chapters, educator quotes and findings were shared to understand the opioid epidemic through the lens of the school. Thus far, the findings focused on educators' voices, lived experiences, and perspectives, shedding light on how the epidemic affects students, schools, and teachers.

This chapter presents the numbers and percentages, highlighting the significance of data gathered from interviews, surveys, and documents. It compiles and visualizes the insights from earlier chapters through graphs, visuals, and tables. The analysis unveils compelling statistics: 97% (n = 28) of interviewees note that students arrive at school without their basic needs met, while 93% (n = 62) of surveyed educators encounter students facing neglect. Remarkably, all interview participants (100%, N = 29) highlight the impact of parental instability. Additionally, 85% (n = 58) of survey respondents report students being removed from home due to a family member's addiction, and 87% (n = 58) have students living with relatives other than parents due to addiction issues.

This research emphasized that children affected by the opioid crisis endure trauma and the strains of household instability, and according to educators, all of which can be linked to their household and environmental exposure to substance abuse and its consequences. The resulting toxic stress often impedes a child's learning process and ability to develop appropriate

DOI: 10.4324/9781003378204-14

social skills, potentially leading to long-term health issues, according to the ACE study (Centers for Disease Control and Prevention, 2014).

Here are the significant findings based on the collection of data.

Significant Findings: Survey Results and Interview Themes

Interviews and open-response questions were coded using Saldana's (2016) coding parameters and methods. As mentioned in Chapter 4, in all 29 interviews and 67 open-ended survey questions, three coding cycles were utilized – *in vivo* coding was the first cycle, followed by descriptive coding, and finally, pattern coding. Particular themes emerged after the three coding cycles, and codes were distributed in categories. Categories were then arranged by superordinate and subordinate measures to focus the investigation's parameters on finding the core and answering each specific research question.

After conducting the multiple rounds of coding, a select number of dominant themes emerged based on the research questions. The emerging dominant themes addressed the following research question: How is the opioid epidemic impacting elementary schools in opioid-crisis regions?

All themes discussed in more than 50% of the 29 interviews are highlighted in Table 11.1. The table outlines the percentages and number (*N*) of participating educators who reported that the opioid epidemic was impacting their classrooms.

As shown in the table, educators reported that the epidemic is impacting their schools through student exposure to drug activity, students coming to

Table 11.1 Interview Themes

Interview Themes of Initial Study	*Mentioned by Participants*	
	%	*N*
Student exposure to drug activity	100	29
Basic needs not met	97	28
Neglect	97	28
Transiency	97	28
Attendance	97	28
Poverty/homelessness	97	28
Student behaviors/NAS behaviors	100	29
Family/parental instability	100	29
Parent behaviors	100	29
Teacher impact/secondary trauma/teacher retention	79	23
Academic impact	65	19

school with unmet basic needs, and neglect. More than 50% of the interview participants also mentioned transiency, attendance, poverty, homelessness, student behaviors, family and parental instability, parent behaviors, secondary teacher trauma, and academic impact as significant indications that the opioid epidemic was impacting their schools, which are located in opioid-crisis regions at the time of this study.

Additionally, in Table 11.2, 67 educators who participated in the survey reported encountering students with various challenging experiences. The percentage and number of participating educators who encountered student experiences directly related to the opioid epidemic are highlighted in Table 11.2. It should be noted that only experiences that yielded 50% or higher are highlighted and shared. Survey participants reported that they witnessed students who experienced neglect, abuse, death of loved ones, removal from home, observed overdoses, born with Neonatal Abstinence Syndrome (NAS), and were involved with the Department of Youth Services.

In addition to reported student experiences, educators also reported a collection of observable behaviors of students who were impacted by the opioid epidemic. The behaviors and challenges listed in Table 11.3 are directly linked to the literature, which reports that prenatal heroin and opioid exposure can be associated with language weaknesses, cognition deficiencies, and attention/hyperactivity disorder. Exposure to opioids contributes to the high occurrence of neurodevelopmental and behavioral problems seen in children in later life (Beckwith & Burke, 2015; Fill et al., 2018; McGlone & Mactier, 2015; Nygaard et al., 2015; Ornoy et al., 2010; Yuan et al., 2014). These behaviors and challenges are not limited to children born with Neonatal Abstinence Syndrome but also to children born into any family battling addiction. Since living in a household with substance addiction is considered an adverse childhood experience (ACE), children living in opioid-abusing households could experience adverse outcomes from disrupted

Table 11.2 Student Experiences Encountered by Survey Participants

Survey Participants – Student Experiences	*%*	*N*
Neglect	93	62
Physical abuse	52	38
Verbal abuse	76	51
Death of parent	56	38
Observed an overdose	51	34
Born with NAS	59	40
Removal from home because of an addicted family member	85	57
Living with a relative other than a parent as a result of addiction	87	58
Placed in foster care	68	46
Department of Youth and Family Service Involvement	79	53

Table 11.3 Behaviors and Challenges Reported by Educators

Survey Participant's Reported Student Behaviors and Challenges	%	N
Sad	88	59
Angry	87	58
Hyperactivity	78	52
Unmotivated	78	52
Cognitive challenges or delays	73	49
Motor challenges or delays	58	38
Behavioral challenges	93	62
Speech, language, and communication disabilities or delays	65	43
Emotional/social challenges	85	56
Poor executive functioning	80	53
Anxiety	84	56

neurodevelopment, including emotional, social, and behavioral disabilities as well as challenges in cognitive and academic functioning (Crouch, 2019). The risk for poor emotional and behavioral outcomes among children living with a parent with a substance abuse history is reported in the literature.

Literature also suggests developmental challenges in children and adolescents living with heroin-addicted mothers, even if the children were not born exposed to opioids *in utero* (Herranz et al., 2014; Nunes et al., 2015). Additionally, research has shown that chaotic and stressful environments, such as living in a home with substance abuse, can inhibit executive functioning development, and that environments lacking healthy parent–child relationships can dampen the development of executive capacities (Barkley, 2001; Evans & Wachs, 2010). Traumatic or prolonged exposure to stress, such as family substance abuse, can lead to toxic stress and can change the architecture of a child's developing brain in ways that can have lasting effects on physiological, cognitive, behavioral, and psychological functioning (Juster et al., 2010; McEwen & Gianaros, 2010).

Based on the literature and the potential behavior and challenges, the participant's experiences align with the noted behaviors and challenges that could potentially be evident in children living in a home or environment with substance abuse, experiencing ACEs, or being born with NAS.

The survey results in Table 11.3 show the percentage of participating educators and the number (*N*) of participating educators who encountered student behaviors and challenges directly related to the disabilities outlined in the literature on exposure to opioid use. In addition to the literature, educators claimed that the behaviors are directly related to community, environmental, and household substance use. It should be noted that only behaviors and challenges that yielded 50% or higher are shared. Survey participants reported that they have witnessed students who are anxious, sad, angry, and hyper with low motivation. Participants also reported that students had cognitive, motor, language, emotional, and executive functioning challenges.

The participants attributed the behaviors and challenges to the impact of the opioid epidemic. However, although the behaviors align with the literature and previously available data, further investigations and additional research would be needed to confirm the educators' assumptions that the behaviors are directly linked to the consequences of the epidemic. Table 11.3 shares reported behaviors and challenges by the educators working in opioid-crisis regions.

In addition to reported student behaviors and challenges, Figure 11.1 organizes the data and findings to emphasize patterns. Figure 11.1 illustrates the impact the opioid epidemic has on schools located in opioid-crisis regions based on the perspectives and data provided by the participating educators.

Using the ACE study as a framework for this research, specifically in understanding the phenomenon of the opioid epidemic and its relationship with the needs of the students born affected/living with environmental influences of this epidemic, Figure 11.1 is a generalization that explicitly illustrates that a selection of ACEs, along with environmental and community factors, are impacting the functions of the school. The visual represents schools in opioid-impacted communities, showing the influence of outside factors that can impact the daily functions of the school.

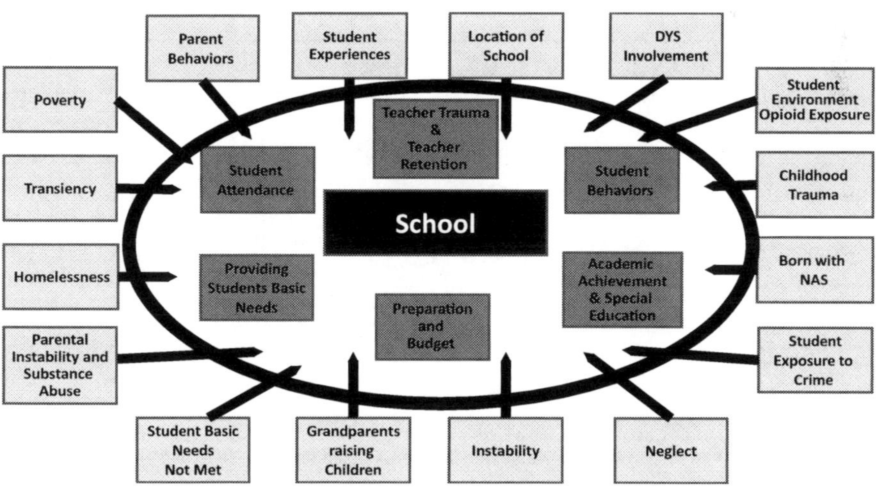

Figure 11.1 Schools located in opioid-impacted communities, highlighting environmental, household, and community influences that impact the functions of the school

As demonstrated in Figure 11.1, the light gray rectangles on the outer area of the diagram represent the outside environment, ACEs, and community factors that influence the function and impact of the schools. Everything inside the oval represents the school community, and the associated specific school impact mentioned by participants is emphasized in the dark gray rectangles. Such impacts mentioned throughout the investigation include preparation and budgets, providing students with necessities needed to address the lack of basic needs met, the impact of student behaviors, student attendance, increased teacher trauma and a possible decrease in teacher retention, and impact on special education and academic achievement.

With all of this impacting the schools, what are the schools doing to prepare educators for the increase of students that are impacted by the challenges related to the opioid epidemic?

Professional Development

Let's reconsider the research question: How are schools in opioid-crisis regions developing and implementing professional development for administrators, teachers, and school staff to address the needs of students impacted by the opioid crisis? In a general report, the schools investigated did not provide professional development specific to the opioid epidemic. However, a percentage of teachers were trained in possible disabilities that can be associated with children born with NAS, living in a household with substance abuse, and children experiencing ACEs. Table 11.4 outlines training

Table 11.4 Teacher Training

Possible Disability Associated With NAS and/or ACEs	*Survey Participants Trained – Prepared*	
	%	*N*
Behavioral disorders	53	35
ADHD	29	19
Cognitive disabilities	45	30
Social-emotional disabilities	73	48
Experienced trauma	83	52
Mental illness, including psychiatric disorders	25	16
Possible situation associated with opioid epidemic exposure		
NAS/living in an opioid-addicted household	8	5
Educators who know what NAS is	30	20
Educators who understand the disabilities associated with NAS	21	14

received by teachers according to the 67 survey participants: 79% (*n* = 52) of teachers had training in trauma, while only 25% (*n* = 16) had training specifically addressing mental illness.

The above chart highlights that educators have had some training on possible disabilities associated with NAS and ACEs. However, there is a lack of professional development specific to the opioid epidemic and NAS. The chart shows that only 8% (*n* = 5) of participants were trained on NAS, 30% (*n* = 20) know what NAS is, and 21% (*n* = 14) understand disabilities associated with NAS.

Bringing It All Together

Returning to the ACE study, key discoveries reveal that the opioid epidemic's persistent influence on students – including environmental, communal, and household exposure – directly impacts the schools. The impacts include influence on educators, student attendance, budget allocations, curriculum, special education referrals, and intervention needs, administrative strategies, and the pivotal role of schools in addressing unmet student needs. Chapter 11 highlights significant findings from interviews, surveys, and documented data, employing graphs, tables, and visual aids to explain the findings. Results highlight key interview themes mentioned in more than 50% of the 29 interviews, calibrated survey results that combine the results of all three case studies, reported student behaviors, educator's preparedness, and described professional development opportunities. Research questions were answered, showing that the epidemic's impact on schools is immediate and intense, and there is a lack of proactive preparation explicitly focusing on professional development to prepare educators for the future of this growing crisis.

References

Barkley, R. A. (2001). The executive functions and self-regulation: An evolutionary neuropsychological perspective. *Neuropsychology Review*, *11*(1), 1–29. https://doi.org/10.1023/A:1009085417776

Beckwith, A. M., & Burke, S. A. (2015). Identification of early developmental deficits in Infants with prenatal heroin, methadone, and other opioid exposure. *Clinical Pediatrics*, *54*(4), 328.

Centers for Disease Control and Prevention. (2014). *The ACE pyramid*. National Center for Injury Prevention and Control, Division of Violence Prevention. https://www.cdc.gov/violenceprevention/acestudy/about.html

Crouch, E., Radcliff, E., Hung, P., & Bennett, K. (2019). Challenges to school success and the role of adverse childhood experiences. *Academic Pediatrics*, *19*(8), 899–907. https://doi-org.proxy3.noblenet.org/10.1016/j.acap.2019.08.006

Evans, G. W., & Wachs, T. D. (Eds.). (2010). *Chaos and its influence on children's development: An ecological perspective*. American Psychological Association. https://doi.org/10.1037/12057-000

Fill, M. A., Miller, A. M., Wilkinson, R. H., Warren, M. D., Dunn, J. R., Schaffner, W., & Jones, T. F. (2018). Educational disabilities among children born with neonatal abstinence syndrome. *Pediatrics*, *142*(3), e20180562. https://doi.org/10.1542/peds.2018-0562

Herranz, G. S., Vílchez, M. A. L., Ledo, J. D., & Sierra, A. M. (2014). Children born to heroin-addicted mothers: What's the outcome 25 years later? *Journal of Addiction Research and Therapy*, *5*(180).

Juster, R. P., McEwen, B. S., & Lupien, S. J. (2010). Allostatic load biomarkers of chronic stress and impact on health and cognition. *Neuroscience and Biobehavioral Reviews*, *35*(1), 2–16. https://doi.org/10.1016/j.neubiorev.2009.10.002

McEwen, B. S., & Gianaros, P. J. (2010). Central role of the brain in stress and adaptation: Links to socioeconomic status, health, and disease. *Annals of the New York Academy of Sciences*, *1186*, 190–222. https://doi.org/10.1111/j.1749-6632.2009.05331.x

McGlone, L., & Mactier, H. (2015). Infants of opioid-dependent mothers: Neurodevelopment at six months. *Early Human Development*, *91*(1), 19–21.

Nunes, E., Weissman, M., Goldsten, R., McAvay, G., Beckford, C., Seracini, A., & Wickramaratne, P. (2015). Psychiatric disorders and impairment in the children of opiate addicts: Prevalence and distribution by ethnicity. *American Journal on Addictions*, *9*(3), 232–241.

Nygaard, E., Moe, V., Slinning, K., & Walhoyd, K. (2015). Longitudinal cognitive development of children born to mothers with opioid and polysubstance use. *Pediatric Research*, *78*(3), 330–335.

Ornoy, A., Daka, L., Goldzweig, G., Gil, Y., Mjen, L., Levit, S., Shufman, E., Bar-Hamburger, R., & Greenbaum, C. (2010). Neurodevelopmental and psychological assessment of adolescents born to drug-addicted parents: Effects of SES and adoption. *Child Abuse & Neglect*, *34*(5), 354–368.

Saldana, J. (2016). *The coding manual for qualitative researchers*. Sage Publications Inc.

Yuan, Q., Rubic, M., Seah, J., Rae, C., Wright, I. M., Kaltenbach, K., Feller, J. M., Abdel-Latif, M. E., Chu, C., & Oei, J. L. (2014). Do maternal opioids reduce neonatal regional brain volumes? A pilot study. *Journal of Perinatology*, *34*(12), 909–913. https://doi.org/10.1038/jp.2014.111

12 Follow-Up Investigations

Post-Pandemic Realities in Schools Located in Opioid-Crisis Regions

> The global pandemic and the opioid epidemic are two forces that have entirely overwhelmed our schools – imagine a child dealing with parental substance abuse, neglect, possible abuse, and food insecurity. School is their safe place, and then suddenly, overnight, your safe place is no longer available for 8, 9, or even 12 months – or they have a "hybrid" safe place- you can imagine the devastation and overwhelming fear that child must have. Now imagine the fear and stress the teachers have when that child is no longer showing up for remote classes and home visits are not allowed. You are probably wondering, "How did we sleep at night?" We did not! This was not one or two students in my class we are talking about here; this was the majority because 95% of our children are in crisis.
>
> – Jolie, New Hampshire Second-Grade Teacher

In 2020, just a few months after the research study's conclusion, schools across the United States closed down because of the COVID-19 global pandemic. This forced a sudden and significant shift in the education system for millions of students, transitioning from traditional, in-person classes to mandatory closures that necessitated remote learning from home.

Historically, public health emergencies and economic and environmental challenges contribute to health and economic disparities, which can, subsequently, be linked to risk factors for child maltreatment (Conrad-Hiebner & Byram, 2020; Wong et al., 2021), adding to the challenges the opioid epidemic have already created in schools. The COVID-19 public health emergency compounds the existing challenges already posed by the opioid epidemic within schools. With the closure of schools, there arose heightened concerns about social isolation and educators' ability to identify instances of child neglect and abuse. Unfortunately, the convergence of the COVID-19 pandemic and the ongoing opioid crisis only amplified these worries. Concerns for children who were experiencing traumas and other challenges were exacerbated, given the number of adverse childhood experiences (ACEs) children in opioid-crisis regions have potentially been exposed

DOI: 10.4324/9781003378204-15

to and are experiencing. Now, they no longer have in-person school to escape to. Consequently, this subsequent investigation revealed many post-pandemic concerns educators experienced in all three case-study locations.

Chapter 12 shares information and data collected from a 2023 follow-up reinvestigation of the three original case-study locations. Seventeen educators from the original study share perspectives and post-pandemic updates. Of those 17 who agreed to participate in the follow-up study, 13 agreed to an interview.

2023 Case-Study Follow-Up and Updates – Maine, Massachusetts, and New Hampshire

School closures have a ripple-down effect on children, particularly children who view school as their safe haven away from the household, community, and environmental impacts that stem from exposure to the opioid epidemic. The COVID-19 pandemic and associated responses, such as school and workplace closures, distancing measures, mandatory isolation, and elevated health risks, negatively impacted mental health (Brannen et al., 2023; Dubey et al., 2020; Horigian et al., 2021; Kola, 2020; Robinson & Daly, 2021). The challenges were exacerbated by already prevalent ACEs from community and household substance abuse and exposure. Opportunities for educators to monitor psychosocial needs, food insecurity, medical, dental, and possible household neglect and abuse were no longer an option, leading to additional challenges and adversity for an already-vulnerable population of children. Given the findings from the research shared in previous chapters, it is pivotal to revisit the schools to understand the impact.

In 2023, each of the three schools were revisited, and the 29 original interview participants and the 67 survey participants from the 2018–2019 study were invited to participate in a follow-up 2023 check-in investigation. The purpose of the follow-up study was to investigate the situation, progress, and proposed solutions outlined in the previous chapters while also developing an understanding of the impact the 2020–2021 school closures had on the schools located in opioid-crisis regions.

Interestingly, out of the original 29 interview participants, only 11 (37.9%) still worked in the same school as in the original study. Additionally, out of the 111 people who qualified to participate in the 2018–2019 initial study, only 44 educators (39.6%) still worked in the three combined districts in 2023. Of those 44 educators, 17 agreed (37.6%) to participate in a follow-up study, 17 completed the qualitative survey, and 13 out of 17 agreed to a follow-up interview. Five participants chose only to complete the survey and did not agree to participate in the interview.

The people who agreed to be interviewed were aware of the previous research because all 13 were interviewed in the original study. Two of the 13 educators changed jobs during this follow-up study and no longer worked in their original school, yet they still agreed to a follow-up interview. Those two participants were also interviewed in the original study. Of the 13 follow-up interview participants, four worked in Massachusetts, four in New Hampshire, three in Maine, and the two who changed schools during the study were previous employees in Massachusetts and New Hampshire. The follow-up study included insight from 13 of the 29 original interview participants (44.8%). By the ninth interview, saturation was reached, and the same familiar patterns and themes were repeated constantly; however, due to an established rapport from the original study and professional curiosity, all 13 interviews were concluded.

Here is the breakdown of the interview findings and updates by school.

Maine Updates

Results were similar to the findings shared in previous chapters. The findings indicated that the Fox Hollow United School still had not provided professional development on the opioid epidemic and the impacts of Neonatal Abstinence Syndrome (NAS), and educators still did not feel prepared to teach children impacted by the epidemic. The only training for educators mentioned by participants was Narcan administration training. Participants also reported that challenges from the COVID-19 pandemic amplified trauma, attendance, food insecurity, secondary teacher trauma, and truancy challenges that the school was already experiencing. Additional challenges included teacher shortages and academic delays due to prolonged school closures. Except extreme teacher shortages and increased academic gaps, findings were similar to the original study. However, some findings highlighted positive solutions, such as a school closure due to location and Maine's Opioid Response Strategic Action Plan that incorporated the school's needs in a community action plan.

Maine has had several updates since the conclusion of the 2019 study. One of the notable updates was that the special education school associated with Fox Hollow United School closed due to its unsafe location. According to a special education teacher, "Students are no longer educated in an area with active drug dealings and drug use. The other areas have it around but at least they are not as obvious." The students were disseminated and transferred to other schools within the district to safer neighborhoods.

Additionally, a Maine administrator explained that Maine has a strategic action plan to combat the opioid epidemic, and although it was in its infancy stages, it brought hope to schools. The administrator explained that the government and community have finally acknowledged that "adverse childhood events, poverty, housing insecurity, and stress impact schools and play a role in the opioid epidemic." He continued to explain that there will be increased investments in the opioid epidemic response to schools. He referred to the Maine Opioid Response: 2023–2025 Strategic Action Plan (2023).

Follow-up research into this plan indicated promising solutions incorporating various community partnerships. The action plan used a multiple-sector approach to decrease the adverse health, public, and economic impact of opioid-use disorders on individuals, families, and communities by focusing on infrastructure, prevention, public safety, harm reduction, treatment, and recovery.

Further investigation based on a copy of the plan indicated the focus area of prevention appeared to address school needs, specifically, "Priority B: Reduce the percentage of Mainers who develop a substance use disorder." Under this priority, there were six goals or strategies to address the area of prevention. The strategies were labeled 7–12, and a brief snapshot of each strategy is explained below (Maine Opioid Response: 2023–2025 Strategic Action Plan, 2023):

Strategy #7: Support healthy early childhood development by ensuring access to Pre-K for every child in Maine to support early childhood development and the prevention of early use of addictive substances. Provide education and training opportunities for childcare providers, promote educational opportunities for parents to develop effective parenting skills, and support social-emotional learning.

Strategy #8: Reduce adverse childhood experiences by promoting awareness and education on childhood brain development and substance-use disorder to high-risk communities and families while developing cross-departmental plans to address ACEs and trauma-informed interventions. Support parents with substance-use disorders in maintaining custody or achieving reunification. Increase the opportunities for deflection from the criminal justice system to avoid trauma from the incarceration of a parent.

Strategy #9: Expand behavioral health support, life skills, and resilience-building capacity and programming for all youth in schools by establishing a primary prevention program in every school in Maine. Also, prioritizing resources and expanding partnerships to address mental health needs, such as including behavioral health counselors in every school and supporting youth in school-based leadership, peer support, and employment opportunities.

Strategy #10: Support policies and initiatives designed to prevent the early use of addictive substances by youth and young adults by reducing youth access to tobacco, alcohol, and cannabis, educating families and communities on the risks and impacts of early use of substances, support public education campaigns, and require proper warning messages at point of sale for all retail license holders.

Strategy #11: Expand local partnerships that educate and engage youth, families, and communities in primary prevention initiatives to include all Maine communities through hosting educational events on best practice prevention policies, support community youth organizations, engage communities in efforts to improve social norms, and establish peer-led programs that support youth impacted by substance-use disorder in their families.

Strategy #12: Invest in secondary prevention efforts that identify and support youth at higher risk for developing a substance-use disorder by providing trauma-informed training to high-risk schools, support restorative justice practices in schools, recruit and train additional instructors for interventions, support the federally funded pediatric and behavioral health tele-consult, and increase the number of behavioral counselors.

As explained, this plan was in the early stages of implementation with a goal that in 2026, every school in Maine would have a primary prevention program.

The Fox Hollow United School and the entire school district are experiencing a significant teacher shortage. Particularly, there is a dire need for special education teachers to the extent that district leaders are spending an abundant time working to bring in new employees, even looking out of state, while the current special education teachers and program leaders are struggling to complete expected tasks such as data collection and developing individualized education programs. As the schools contend with the aftermath of the COVID-19 pandemic and the ongoing opioid crisis in the regions, they are tasked with redoing their special education programs and initiatives to work for the minimal staff they have.

In conclusion, Maine's Fox Hollow United is experiencing the same challenges as the original study. However, some challenges worsened because of the consequences of the COVID-19 school closures, such as trauma, chronic absenteeism, food insecurity, secondary teacher trauma, response from the Department of Youth Services, and truancy – challenges the school was already experiencing. New challenges included teacher shortages and academic delays from gaps in schooling due to the pandemic school closures. On a positive note, the school that was located amid drug activity has closed, disseminating all students to another district school in safer neighborhoods. Additionally, Maine created an opioid response action plan that includes the community schools with a goal that in 2026, every school in Maine will have a primary prevention program.

New Hampshire Updates

Similar to Maine, New Hampshire participants reported that challenges from the aftermath of the COVID-19 pandemic have amplified trauma, anxiety, attendance, food insecurity, secondary teacher trauma, and truancy challenges the school was already experiencing. The 2023 findings were similar to the 2018–2019 study. Changes since the original study included teacher and leadership turnover and drastic increases in special education percentages. On a positive note, there was an additional position to highlight – a community liaison.

One notable change is that the number of students who attended the Cobbs Hill School who received special education services increased from 16% in 2018 to 20% in 2023. The participants in the original case study predicted this increase due to the 2019–2020 numbers of incoming kindergarten students with significant needs. Furthermore, considering the increase of children with disabilities, special education teacher shortages are a concern at the school. According to participants, current special education teacher caseloads are exceedingly high, sometimes over 26 students per teacher as compared to ten or so students per teacher back in 2019. Special education teachers' caseloads have doubled, while many special educators are leaving the profession, transferring schools, and leaving the New Hampshire school district. According to a K-2 special educator:

> Combining the effects of the opioid epidemic and the COVID-19 pandemic is just crushing our resources. We try so hard, but there are too many students with double the needs, double the trauma, double the behaviors, and . . . it is just. My heart is broken. We do not have enough people, not enough special education teachers, not enough mental health providers, not enough resources to help the children here. We cannot find someone to take this on and lead our school. I do not have answers, but I can no longer be a part of this. I am failing these kids. I, too, will be leaving this school and possibly this career – hopefully by January. It is not fair to my family. I bring home too much of this pain.

Since the original case study in 2019, the Cobbs Hill School has experienced significant leadership and staff turnover. From 2019 to 2023, four different principals have come and left, and consequently, this has resulted in teacher turnover. According to a second-grade teacher, "all the trauma-informed initiatives, mental health initiatives, Toolbox Projects, and school-wide programs change as the administration changes." She added, "There is no follow-through, and systems continue to break down." According to a former special education teacher at the Cobbs Hill School, "Leaders are hired to turn the school around, fail quickly, and leave soon after. Which is creating chaos in an already chaotic situation." She continued, "You feel bad for the students you are leaving, but it is a deteriorating situation. It is hard to be part of this and watch our students hurt." Another participant added, "The district is trying. They are even hiring administrators who are famous, write books, and are known to turn schools around, but I guess we were just too much for them because even that one left." Leadership turnover was mentioned as the reason for teacher turnover and continued disarray in the Cobbs Hill School.

Additionally, participants shared that the response time for the Department of Youth Services continues to be delayed. However, new school-wide systems (post-pandemic) were in place to try to minimize the lost students. Even with systems in place, an uptick in chronic absenteeism makes it difficult for staff to track missing students.

According to participants, students were lost, unaccounted for, and went missing during remote learning. When students went missing, they would eventually be unenrolled. Nevertheless, as mentioned by seven participants (from both New Hampshire and Massachusetts), New Hampshire and Massachusetts faced a horrible situation, The Harmony Montgomery Case. In 2019, a young girl, Harmony Montgomery, went missing. However, it was not reported until two years later. She was lost within the system and unaccounted for. Unfortunately, the girl was allegedly murdered by her father. It was a case of a mother and father who were dealing with the challenges of substance abuse. The father, who was known to law enforcement agencies, also had a history of crime and incarceration. Parental struggles and a collection of failures of various child protection systems to protect and keep track of Harmony ended in devastation (Office of Child Advocate, 2022). Since this case unfolded, New Hampshire schools have been trying to improve tracking of students and not unenroll students until a parent or guardian unenrolls them. Unfortunately, participants still were frustrated with the lack of response from the Department of Youth Services when children were lost or abused. The Harmony Montgomery Case was mentioned and referred to by participants as a reason why the Department of Youth Services needs to respond quickly. According to a former New Hampshire educator:

> I am sure you have heard of the Harmony Montgomery Case. Honestly, I cannot stop thinking about it because that literally could have been any of my students. Any of my students that I repeatedly called DCYF and waited for help, and most of the time, I got nothing . . . no help. I was sending kids home to families like that, and I could not sleep at night and just prayed that they would be back in school tomorrow. And then the pandemic hit in the middle of all that, and those students were home every day dealing with situations that I cannot even talk to you about today – I had enough. I was so angry every day. I felt hopeless.

Another participant explained, "The system continues to fail students and children suffering – did you read about the horrible Harmony case? . . . That is too close to the type of stuff we experience. The story hits too close to home."

Cobbs Hill School has tried to take matters into its own hands and started a new community liaison position to keep track of students and serve as a "middle person" between the school and families. The community liaison is a known member of the neighborhood community, is known to the school's families, and hopes to strengthen the community, families, educators, and schools.

In conclusion, from the perspectives of the educators, New Hampshire's Cobbs Hill School appeared to be in a difficult situation but was trying to establish more consistent leadership to address the challenges they were facing. Each leader who stepped in to address the issue failed and left. Participants explained that each new leader brought their own solutions and disregarded their predecessor's attempts, causing chaos in an already-chaotic school. In addition, participants reported that challenges from the COVID-19 pandemic amplified trauma, anxiety, attendance, food insecurity, secondary teacher trauma, DYS responses, and truancy challenges the school was already experiencing. The 2023 findings are similar to the 2018–2019 study, with added concerns of leadership turnover, special education teacher shortages, and a drastic increase in students identified as having a disability and needing special education services.

Massachusetts Updates

In agreement with Maine and New Hampshire, Massachusetts participants reported that challenges from the COVID-19 pandemic amplified trauma, anxiety, attendance, food insecurity, secondary teacher trauma, and truancy challenges that the Anderson Loop School was already experiencing because of their location. The findings were similar to the original study. Notable increases in chronic absences were a primary concern post-pandemic for the Anderson Loop School. Another significant challenge post-pandemic was the lack of early interventions, missing identifiers of early trauma from preschool, and shortages of special education teachers and paraprofessionals. Additionally, participants also felt that the response from the Department of Youth Services continued to be a problem of concern, which continuously gets worse with longer responses and turnaround wait times. A Massachusetts assistant principal mentioned that any interventions that were started to address the impact of the opioid epidemic were put on hold because of school closures and the COVID-19 crisis and have yet to be revisited. On a positive note, the attendance/truancy officer was given additional staff to help locate students, and the school hired a family engagement specialist and additional counselors.

According to an Anderson Loop school administrator, chronic absentee rates were around 10% in 2016 and have increased to over 20%. He explained that the pandemic created a critical issue with students not attending school. He said that it is an amplified ramification of COVID-19 school closures in opioid crisis districts because of household substance abuse, trauma, neglect, and abuse, stating that "students absolutely need to be here – in school. They need to be here because we are monitoring their daily status, their functioning, their mental health, and we keep tabs if things are not right." He continued:

> If things are not safe in the household, and they do not come to school, it is not reported, it is overlooked, and it can have devastating consequences. Kids need to come to school. In this community, it is unsafe if they do not show up here.

Another post-pandemic concern for the Anderson Loop School was the gap in early disability evaluations and trauma identification coming from preschool because children were not attending preschool and not receiving early interventions. According to the assistant principal, "It is a challenge when the children come to use without attending preschool. Kids are coming to us as just a name on paper, and we are always surprised at the level of need, trauma, behaviors, and disabilities." He continued to explain that they cannot proactively staff for the student's needs. Identifying and obtaining the needed services for the children can sometimes take up to 24 weeks. Chronic absenteeism and uninvolved parents are adding to the situation, resulting in children falling through the cracks. He and others mentioned that there appeared to be a drastic increase in children who have disabilities, behavior challenges, and social-emotional needs. He attributed this to the opioid epidemic, children born with NAS, and the ramifications of the COVID-19 pandemic. Further investigation into the publicly available data through the Massachusetts Department of Education confirmed that the number of students who attended the Anderson Loop School with a disability and received special education services increased from 10% in 2018 to over 18% in 2023. Again, this is a confirmed educator's prediction from the original study.

In conclusion, all the initiatives that were started to address the needs of the students impacted by the opioid crisis were put on hold to address the ramifications of the COVID-19 pandemic and have yet to be revisited. It was discovered that challenges from the COVID-19 pandemic amplified trauma, anxiety, attendance, food insecurity, secondary teacher trauma, and truancy challenges that the Anderson Loop School was already experiencing because of its opioid crisis location. The findings were similar to the original study. Notable increases in chronic absences were a primary concern post-pandemic for the Anderson Loop School. Another significant challenge post-pandemic was the lack of early interventions, missing identifiers of early trauma from preschool, and shortages of special education teachers and paraprofessionals.

Post-Pandemic Similarities Between the Schools

Results indicated that all three case-study sites have not provided professional development on the opioid epidemic and the impacts of NAS, and educators still do not feel prepared to teach children impacted by the epidemic. Interview participants also reported that challenges from the COVID-19 pandemic have amplified trauma (n = 12), attendance (n = 10), food insecurity (n = 11), secondary teacher trauma (n = 11), and transiency challenges (n = 10) the school was already experiencing. Also, 100% (n = 13) mentioned challenges with and no improvements in the response of the Department of Youth Services. This continues to be an extremely frustrating challenge for all three schools, causing educator distress and secondary trauma. Those challenges parallel the original finding discussed in earlier chapters, and, unfortunately, educators have not perceived or reported improvements. Some notable and additional challenges in all three locations were an increase in chronic absenteeism mentioned by 100% (N = 13) of participants, 69% (n = 9) mentioned leadership turnover, and 69% (n = 9) mentioned teacher shortages. Post-pandemic challenges were even more complex, pertinent, and challenging in opioid-crisis regions.

Investigating further chronic absenteeism and post-pandemic schooling, chronic absenteeism rates were a national concern. According to the United States Department of Education, chronic absenteeism means missing at least 10% of days in a school year for any reason, including excused and unexcused absences. Specifically, according to reports on Attendance Works (2023), a nationally available database, Massachusetts, New Hampshire, and Maine's chronic absentee numbers increased dramatically from pre- to post-pandemic. In 2019, 12.80% (n = 122,242) of students in Massachusetts were chronically absent, compared to 27.80% (n = 252,976) in 2022. New Hampshire and Maine were experiencing similar situations, reinforcing educator's post-pandemic opioid-crisis region worries. In 2019, 13% (n = 23,243) of students in New Hampshire were chronically absent, compared to 33.30% (n = 56,427) in 2022. Similarly, in 2019, Maine had 16.40% (n = 29,601) of students chronically absent, compared to 30.90% (n = 53,574) in 2022. All three states had at least a 100% increase in chronic absenteeism. Chronic absenteeism is an amplified challenge because of household substance abuse and household trauma, neglect, and abuse. Going to school is critical in crisis regions because educators monitor students' moods, behaviors, physical appearance, and mental health. If students do not show up, situations may not be reported or go unnoticed, leading to potentially stressful and horrifying consequences.

The other complicated issue all three locations elaborated on was teacher shortages and leadership turnover. From 2019 to 2023, it was clear that when revisiting each location, there was vast turnover. Leadership, staff, and faculty changes were evident. Consequently, reaching out to the 29 original interview participants and finding that only 11 were still working in the schools is a significant finding. Trying to make changes and create a state of continuous improvement in a school that is constantly in flux would be challenging, even for the most experienced district leader. Understandably, initiatives were lost in the transition.

Teacher shortages and leadership turnover are a national trend, but the consequences are exacerbated in opioid-crisis regions.

Significant Findings – 2023 Follow-Up Study

Interestingly, only 11 of the 29 interview participants still worked in the school districts of the original study, and, in total, only 44 out of 111 educators remained in their original school district, confirming the educator concerns from 2018 to 2019. Specifically, during the interviews in 2018–2019, 79% of educators mentioned secondary teacher trauma and retention concerns. Consequently, within about 4 years, approximately 61% of the participants left the schools where they were employed in 2019.

Table 12.1 highlights the 2023 interview themes. Many of the same patterns and themes uncovered in 2018–2019 were reintroduced by participants in the 2023 interviews and are listed in the table. For example, 100%

Table 12.1 Interview Themes – 2023 Follow-Up Study

Interview Themes of 2023 Follow-Up Study	*Mentioned by Participants*	
	%	*N*
Student exposure to drug activity	100	13
Basic needs not met/food insecurity	84	11
Trauma/ACEs	92	12
Neglect	76	10
Transiency	76	10
Attendance/chronic absenteeism	100	13
Department of Youth Services	100	13
Poverty/homelessness	84	11
Teacher shortages	69	9
Leadership turnover	69	9
Student behaviors	53	7
Family/parental instability	100	13
Increase in disabilities/special education	92	12
Teacher impact/secondary trauma/teacher retention	84	11
Loss of learning/academic gap	84	11

of participants discussed exposure, attendance concerns, Department of Youth Services, and family instability. There were a few additional concerns, such as teacher shortages and leadership turnover, mentioned by 69% of participants. Increased special education needs were mentioned by 92%, and post-COVID academic gaps were mentioned by 84%. The other categories and themes are shared in Table 12.1.

As mentioned above, interview saturation was achieved by the ninth interview. However, all 13 of the educators who volunteered were interviewed. The conversations were remarkably similar to the initial study highlighted in previous chapters – different stories, yet the same concerns with a few additional themes. Because the findings were so similar, it was essential to explore external validity and whether the findings of this study could be extended.

External Validity Study

The initial case-study investigation was in 2018–2019. The research was repeated to uncover updates in the same three schools four years later in 2023, and the findings, themes, and patterns proved similar. To demonstrate reliability, it was important to explore external validity and whether the findings of this study could be extended to other locations and schools. In other words, can the results of this multiple-case study be generalized across similar but different geographic locations across the United States?

To confirm or deny the hypothesis that this study would have similar results regardless of geographic location, a third approval from the Internal Review Board (IRB) was necessary. A follow-up study was established by surveying and interviewing educators who worked in multiple qualifying locations to measure reliability. The qualitative study collected educators' perspectives from surveys and interviews from similar school districts in opioid-crisis regions to understand the educators and school lens on the impact the opioid epidemic had on schools.

Sampling

Purposeful sampling was used for the identification and intentional selection of participants who would be considered knowledgeable and have experience working in schools located in opioid-crisis regions. According to Creswell and Plano Clark (2018), purposeful sampling involves identifying and selecting individuals or groups especially knowledgeable about or experienced with a phenomenon of interest. The phenomenon is the impact of the opioid epidemic in schools located in opioid-crisis regions through the lens of the school and the perspectives of the educators working within the schools.

Twenty school districts were identified as having significantly higher overdose rates per 100,000 people than the national average, which is greater than 30 documented overdose deaths per 100,000 people within a year. To qualify, the school district needed similar demographics as the three case study schools. Such demographics included a high-needs district with over 5,000 students with multiple ethnicities, more than 50% of the school qualified for free or reduced lunch, and a high immigration population. It should be noted that throughout the Northeast and, more broadly, the United States, more than 20 districts would qualify.

Within those 20 school districts, four educators per district were randomly, yet purposefully, selected using district staff directories and asked to participate in a survey, the same survey the 2023 case-study participants filled out. One of the four educators selected was an administrator. Eighty survey links were disseminated to educators working in the 20 qualifying school districts. Interview volunteers were also solicited within the survey.

Participants

Of the 80 distributed survey links, 31 educators (38.7%) completed the survey, with 17 educators volunteering to participate in interviews. Fourteen different school districts were represented in the 31 surveys. Nine out of the 17 interviews were completed until saturation was achieved.

There was a decent sample of diverse positions represented: 36% of the participants were elementary education teachers, 23% were administrators, 23% were special education teachers, 7% were specialists, 3% were early childhood educators, and a school counselor and a behavior specialist completed the survey.

Most participants, 83%, had over 15 years of experience, while 17% had less than 15 years of experience.

Method of Analysis

Identical to the analysis of the initial and follow-up study (in-depth method of analysis and coding specifics are shared in Chapter 4), all survey open-ended responses and interviews were transcribed verbatim and coded similarly. Three coding cycles were utilized in all 31 surveys and nine interviews using Saldana (2016) to guide the coding method. In vivo coding was the first cycle, followed by descriptive coding and pattern coding. Specific themes emerged, and after the three coding cycles, codes were distributed in the coding categories. Categories were then arranged by superordinate and subordinate themes. A select number of dominant themes emerged. Patterns and percentages were created based on how frequently the codes emerged in combining all interviews and surveys. It became the dominant theme if a code emerged 50% or more during the combined interviews and surveys.

Findings

According to survey participants, 29 out of 31 participants had students in their class impacted by the opioid epidemic. Of those 29 participants, 100% ($N = 29$) reported that their school district was not preparing for the increase of students impacted, and 86% ($n = 25$) had not had any training or professional development on the opioid epidemic, NAS, or associated disabilities. Fourteen percent ($n = 4$) had some training or knowledge of NAS and associated disabilities, and 56% ($n = 17$) did not feel prepared to teach students impacted by the epidemic. Of the educators surveyed, 93% ($n = 27$) reported that since the COVID-19 pandemic school closures, their students had experienced an increase in trauma.

Interview themes are shared in Table 12.1. The themes outlined were mentioned in 50% or more of the interviews are highlighted in the following.

There are three minor yet notable differences in the 2023 case study updates compared to the 2018–2019 original study. Leadership turnover was mentioned frequently. While student behaviors were mentioned in less than 50% of the interviews in this study. However, instead of behaviors in general, 77% ($n = 7$) mentioned that students were acting "unsocialized," which was a more specific theme than just behaviors. Through further questioning, participants explained that students struggled to adjust to developmentally appropriate social norms and expectations. Many emphasized ramifications from social isolation that impacted students' ability to engage in age-appropriate conversations. Two participants in different districts described students' social isolation and behaviors as "feral." Educators felt that the neglect from parents dealing with substance-abuse disorders and addictions made social isolation worse than that of a student not living in a home or community with substance abuse challenges. Table 12.2 shows the other themes from the follow-up study.

Student exposure and stories related to drug activity, along with trauma, chronic absenteeism, and teacher secondary trauma, were coded in 100% of all interviews. Loss of learning, increased special education needs, neglect, poverty, and stories related to the Department of Youth Services were mentioned and coded in 88% of the interviews. Transiency and the impact of students coming and going, getting lost in the system, or not returning to school were coded in 77% of the interviews. Many districts were experiencing teacher shortages, and many children were faced with food insecurity and unmet basic needs.

Collected quotes are very similar to the original study and follow-up study, and a snapshot sample of voices and perspectives of educators are located in Appendix 12.1.

Table 12.2 Interview Themes – External Validity Study

Interview Themes of 2023 External Validity Study	*Mentioned by Participants*	
	%	*N*
Student exposure to drug activity	100	9
Basic needs not met/food insecurity	66	6
Trauma/ACEs	100	9
Neglect	88	8
Transiency	77	7
Attendance/chronic absenteeism	100	9
Department of Youth Services	88	8
Poverty/homelessness	88	8
Teacher shortages	66	6
Family/parental instability	88	8
Increase in disabilities/special education	88	8
Teacher impact/secondary trauma/teacher retention	100	9
Unsocialized	77	7
Loss of learning/academic gap	88	8

Bringing It All Together

In 2020, the COVID-19 pandemic caused widespread school closures in the United States, prompting a shift from traditional in-person education to remote learning. Revisiting the original three case-study locations highlighted the pandemic's exacerbation of existing challenges such as trauma, attendance issues, food insecurity, teacher distress, and transiency among students. Interviews mirrored earlier findings, underlining common concerns while revealing additional complexities. Interview participants reported that challenges from the COVID-19 pandemic intersecting with the opioid epidemic had amplified trauma (n = 12), attendance (n = 10), food insecurity (n = 11), secondary teacher trauma (n = 11), and transiency challenges (n = 10), which the school was already experiencing. Interview conversations were remarkably similar to the initial study highlighted in previous chapters – different stories, yet the same concerns with a few additional themes. Maine's Opioid Response: Strategic Action Plan was a positive highlight and noteworthy solution that had just begun implementation.

Consistency was established through exploration and a follow-up study to investigate external validity and understand educators' perspectives in additional opioid crisis districts outside the three participating schools, and the results of the case study can be generalized and extended to other locations based on the similarities in interview themes, quotes, and survey results. Based on these findings, it can be concluded that the results of the multiple case studies can be generalized across similar but different geographic locations across the country. It appeared that all locations were struggling with similar challenges. Yet all districts had diverse resources, funding, and autonomy to address the issue the opioid epidemic created in the schools.

References

Attendance Works. (2023). *Rising tide of chronic absence challenges schools*. https://www.attendanceworks.org/rising-tide-of-chronic-absence-challenges-schools/ and supplemental spreadsheet: https://docs.google.com/spreadsheets/d/15yNTUUNwHzhFjQRCYgY5o7KE5pGoVFtk/edit#gid=1137911798

Brannen, D. E., Wynn, S., Shuster, J., & Howell, M. (2023). Pandemic isolation and mental health among children. In J. J. James (Ed.), *Disaster medicine and public health preparedness* (Vol. 17, p. e353). https://doi.org/10.1017/dmp.2023.7

Conrad-Hiebner, A., & Byram, E. (2020). The temporal impact of economic insecurity on child maltreatment: A systematic review. *Trauma, Violence, & Abuse*, *21*(1), 157–178. https://doi.org/10.1177/1524838018756122

Creswell, J. W., & Plano Clark, V. L. (2018). *Designing and conducting mixed methods research* (3rd ed.). SAGE.

Dubey, S., Biswas, P., Ghosh, R., Chatterjee, S., Dubey, M. J., Chatterjee, S., Lahiri, D., & Lavie, C. J. (2020). Psychosocial impact of COVID-19. *Diabetes & Metabolic Syndrome*, *14*(5), 779–788. https://doi.org/10.1016/j.dsx.2020.05.035

Horigian, V. E., Schmidt, R. D., & Feaster, D. J. (2021). Loneliness, mental health, and substance use among U.S. young adults during COVID-19. *Journal of Psychoactive Drugs*, *53*(1), 1–9. https://doi.org/10.1080/02791072.2020.1836435

Kola, L. (2020). Global mental health and COVID-19. *The Lancet Psychiatry*, *7*(8), 655–657.

Maine Opioid Response: 2023–2025 Strategic Action Plan. (2023). *Maine Governor's office of policy innovation and the future*. https://www.maine.gov/future/sites/maine.gov.future/files/2023-08/GOPIF_OpioidReport_2023_exsum_digital_0.pdf

Office of Child Advocate. (2022). *Investigative report: Multisystem investigation regarding Harmony Montgomery*. State Library of Massachusetts. https://archives.lib.state.ma.us/handle/2452/858974

Robinson, E., & Daly, M. (2021). Explaining the rise and fall of psychological distress during the COVID-19 crisis in the United States: Longitudinal evidence from the understanding America study. *British Journal of Health Psychology*, *26*(2), 570–587.

Saldana, J. (2016). *The coding manual for qualitative researchers*. Sage Publications Inc.

Wong, J. Y.-H., Wai, A. K.-C., Wang, M. P., Lee, J. J., Li, M., Kwok, J. Y.-Y., Wong, C. K.-H., & Choi, A. W. M. (2021). Impact of COVID-19 on child maltreatment: Income instability and parenting issues. *International Journal of Environmental Research and Public Health*, *18*(4), 1501. http://dx.doi.org/10.3390/ijerph18041501

Appendix 12.1

A Sampling of Educator Quotes

Here is a random sampling of quotes categorized by topics from the survey and interviews shared by participants within the 14 school districts throughout the Northeast. The quotes and educator's perspectives are similar to those who participated in the multiple case studies. This additional investigation helps confirm external validity.

Secondary Trauma

We have former students dying from opioid use. We've gone to teenagers' funerals for this. That's not normal. You know what I mean? That's really not normal. This is secondary trauma (P1, Personal Communication, October 2023).

Sometimes, I am traumatized because I have to betray a child, even though it's for their own good. They come to me and tell me horrible situations about Mom or Dad shooting up heroin, and there is abuse, neglect, and things I cannot even tell you. Betraying them hurts, but necessary (P3, Personal Communication, October 2023).

Our young teachers are physically and mentally ill because they are in complete shock. Teacher prep needs to prepare teachers for the possibility of secondary trauma (P7, Personal Communication, November 2023).

COVID-19 – School Closures

COVID had the impact of freezing the kids in the horrible places that they needed help from. I'm watching this kid in this home setting, and I can't do anything about it. And DCF pretty much closed down during social isolation, or maybe they just did an even worse job responding to our cries for help . . . who knows? But at least you could be a safe person for them when they were online (P2, Personal Communication, October 2023).

When we were on Zoom, you had a glimpse of a visual into their home life. And so it was difficult to sort out what was normal for a family versus what was concerning. Sometimes, I think, you saw things that were not reportable but concerning (P8, Personal Communication, November 2023).

If you have a kid in a class and all of a sudden they're wearing the same clothes multiple days, or they look like they're tired or whatever, you can check-in. During COVID you could not do that by Zoom. You wouldn't notice it as much when schools were closed. I know a lot was happening, but collecting that evidence was impossible (P1, Personal Communication, October 2023).

Special Education Increases

Because of kids born addicted, special education numbers are going way up, so much so that schools all over are doing something completely illegal . . . they are rewriting kids IEPs to meet the staff they have because of the teacher shortages. Huge no no (P1, Personal Communication, October 2023).

We have so many students with disabilities, many more this year than ever. Many are developmentally challenged because their parents are drug addicted. We also have operational defiance disorder kids. And often, those kids come from households that have opioid drug addiction issues (P9, Personal Communication, November 2023).

I think the biggest thing, and it's hard to determine how much is the epidemic, how much is the pandemic, how much is a combination of the two, and other factors. . . . But we are seeing a disproportional number of kindergartners coming in with significant cognitive and behavioral issues at a much higher rate than we did before the pandemic, but at the same time, in a consistent escalation with the opioid epidemic (P9, Personal Communication, November 2023).

Teacher Turnover/Retention

A big problem with teacher turnover in this district is teachers cannot go back a year or two and get a history on a child that is dealing with parents' opioid-use disorder and trauma because the teacher is gone (P2, Personal Communication, October 2023).

I go home exhausted every night, but knowing I made a difference and it was great, but the mental wear and tear is hard. I cannot see myself here longer than another two years (P7, Personal Communication, November 2023).

We are seeing an incredible rate of burnout. We're losing teachers. This is a very difficult place to work. This is not necessarily an overly desirable place for people. It's not easy to teach in this district, and it certainly has the reputation of such that it's not something that a lot of people seek out (P2, Personal Communication, October 2023).

People are not flocking to teaching anymore. And the challenges that we're facing with students, both due to the opioid crisis and in the aftereffects of the pandemic, are driving people away from the profession (P4, Personal Communication, October 2023).

Chronic Absenteeism

Twenty percent or more of our student population that was chronically absent last year. This year is not going well either (P2, Personal Communication, October 2023).

In a school of 700, we have 70–100 kids who are chronically absent in a given year, and that speaks for itself (P9, Personal Communication, November 2023).

We have a huge chronic absenteeism issue – we did because we are an opioid epicenter, and now it is worse post-remote school. I wonder if others have the same issues we do or if its unique to us (P7, Personal Communication, November 2023).

Department of Youth Services

Our students want to get DCF workers to wear a body camera. And they said, because if your parent's doing bad things, the social worker writes things down. And if they have a relationship with your parent, they won't write down the bad things they're seeing because they want to help the parent not the kids. But if they had a camera, the DCF worker can't lie for the parent. . . . I was like, wow, that's powerful. . . . I say out of the mouths of babes all the time, but sometimes they have answers for things we can't even begin to think about (P1, Personal Communication, October 2023).

I think that the social services, DCF, whatever it's called now, should get a massive infusion of funding so that any reports of neglect and concern are followed up quickly, thoroughly, and reasonably. The hardest part of my job was reporting students to DCF who were in crisis, and nothing was ever done. I felt like I contributed to the abuse because I could not stop it. I was just ignored (P4, Personal Communication, October 2023).

DCF returns students to early parental custody after being in foster care – we would see an immense decline in their well-being. DCF needs a massive overhaul (P7, Personal Communication, November 2023).

During school closures, we got a lot of mixed messages from the Department of Children and Families because they were getting a disproportionate amount of filings for abuse and neglect. DCF was getting overwhelmed with calls, especially in the early and middle months of the pandemic. They were overwhelmed, and we were told to stop filing (P9, Personal Communication, November 2023).

Homelessness/Poverty

Because you can't go into a shelter if you're not 18 and if you don't have a parent, some of these kids run away from home because they're in bad situations with opioid-addicted parents. They try to get out of the situation (P6, Personal Communication, October 2023).

It's shocking how many kids are either couch-surfing or have no home. I'm actually really surprised by that. And I don't even think it's written anywhere. I don't even know if the data is collected anywhere. So some of these kids in these homes where parents are doing drugs, they're escaping, and they're couch-surfing (P2, Personal Communication, October 2023).

There is a very high percentage of homeless students. Just in the last year that I was teaching, we had a couple of students whose parents seemed to be absent from the home and were left with sort of a mishmash of neighbors, friends, and relatives with increasing frequency and without warning. So we had some major concerns (P9, Personal Communication, November 2023).

Professional Development

I don't think if I've ever had any professional development on this (P7, Personal Communication, November 2023).

I don't think I've ever had any. I can't. . . . Unless I'm just not thinking of something. I can't think of ever having any professional development on this (P4, Personal Communication, October 2023).

Not specifically, no. We did have some trauma-based professional development that was more broad based, but very little that was actually specific to opioids (P9, Personal Communication, November 2023).

Is that a serious question, because if it does not involve improving the MCAS scores, we do not have professional development on it. Our district thinks Math and ELA scores are more important than student's mental health and well-being. Actually, that is probably a Massachusetts thing (P4, Personal Communication, October 2023).

Solutions

There are no district-wide solutions, just teachers who care a lot. A teacher in my school started a backpack program a few years ago. We would all bring in donations of food, and then every Friday, she would give students a backpack full of food. So that it would look like everybody else's backpack. And they'd have the food in it. On Monday, they bring a backpack back, and the next Friday, they would have a backpack of food to bring home again (P1, Personal Communication, October 2023).

Our school has free lunch for everyone, medical, and dental visits for kids (P4, Personal Communication, October 2023).

We need a full-time drug counselor, a full-time social worker, and full-time school psychologist – in this district, we cannot afford that, but need that (P6, Personal Communication, October 2023).

We need more mental health support. We need more ability for families to access mental health resources and more services, not just here at school (P7, Personal Communication, November 2023).

I would love for the school day to be longer. I would love for these teachers to be compensated for that longer school day. I would love for there to be funding for buses – I do feel that this is their safe place away from addiction and trauma. I feel like, if some of them could stay here until it was time for bed, they would, but we don't have the busing or funding (P2, Personal Communication, October 2023).

13 Discussion of Theoretical Implications and Associated National Trends

Unraveling the Complex Web of Educational Challenges in Opioid-Crisis Regions

> The teachers are not equipped to deal with the amount of trauma sitting in front of them and they're not supported enough to deal with that. And it's a hard job. It's a hard job in our district because accountability is so high. In a district like this, we are under the microscope all the time. And it's extremely difficult to teach when you have children who are struggling with trauma and needs. Because to those children school does not matter. The trauma that they're dealing with is so much bigger than learning and passing the MCAS. They could care less about school because their world is so shattered. . . . But the state concern is that we need to increase those MCAS scores.
>
> – Richard, Massachusetts Special Education Administrator

There is a profound intersection of adverse childhood experiences (ACEs) and Maslow's hierarchy of needs within the context of students and schools, particularly in regions contending with the opioid epidemic. The educational landscape is experiencing a shift as schools face the daunting task of addressing students' unmet basic needs, safety concerns, and the pervasive impact of trauma on learning. Drawing on Maslow's foundational theory, an intricate web connects students' essential learning and development requirements with the challenges arising from ACEs, and stressors were exacerbated by the COVID-19 pandemic. In highlighting the relationship between Maslow's framework and the ACE study, a narrative emerges – one where students' ability to learn and thrive is intricately linked to providing safety, security, and a sense of belonging. Further discussion illuminates the compounding effects of the opioid crisis, emphasizing the urgent need for schools to address not only academic challenges but also the multifaceted social, emotional, and mental health needs of both students and educators. Furthermore, intricate threads are tying together teacher stress, attrition, and shortages in crisis regions. These issues and challenges are magnified by the opioid crisis and intensified by the aftermath of the COVID-19 pandemic.

DOI: 10.4324/9781003378204-16

As the discussion unfolds and national trends are introduced, it is evident that a comprehensive, collaborative, and multi-tiered approach is imperative to mitigate the far-reaching consequences of the opioid epidemic on the education system. This chapter further sets the stage for a discussion of interventions and solutions crucial for reshaping the future of education in the wake of an ongoing public health emergency.

ACEs Intersect With Maslow – Students and Schools

Students attending school with their basic needs unmet is a consequential situation schools in opioid epidemic crisis areas are experiencing. Safety concerns, food insecurity, and inconsistent living arrangements paired with multiple adverse childhood experiences and trauma can make it extremely difficult to grow, learn, and thrive in school. Students come to school with abundant stress, mental health challenges, lack of necessities, unstable housing, food insecurity, and adverse childhood experiences that impact learning. These concerns have amplified since the COVID-19 pandemic. The ACE study (2014) and Maslow's hierarchy of needs (1968) are theoretical implications of the adaptive challenge. Unfortunately, adverse home and community factors are associated with lost learning opportunities.

Maslow's hierarchy of needs (1968) suggests that only after fulfilling the needs of food, warmth, rest, security, safety, and belonging can a person realize growth or experience learning. Lack of nutrition significantly affects a child's academic gains (Berliner, 2009). Without these basic needs, such as safety and belonging, students will be less apt to engage in academics and learning (Maslow, 1968). Maslow's hierarchy of needs is critical in understanding the potential lack of learning and achievement in opioid-crisis regions. As the research found, not only are children coming to school hungry and tired, but they are also unable to focus on academic requirements. Immediate basic needs for safety, security, and belonging are not being met because of potentially toxic stress in the community and at home.

In conjunction with Maslow's theory, the ACE study (2014) added another layer of complication, citing that adverse childhood experiences are major risk factors for the leading causes of illness, disability, death, and poor quality of life in the United States. Higher opioid prescription, usage, and mortality rates have been linked with an increased risk of child abuse, neglect, and accidental injury (Drescher et al., 2022), all considered adverse childhood experiences. When combining the unmet basic needs from Maslow's theory and the outcomes of the ACE study, it is evident that the impact on school and learning is magnified.

Daily exposure to the opioid crisis and the effects of exposure directly impact a student's ability to come to school and learn. The ramifications of adverse childhood experiences and unmet needs influence schools in crisis regions. Schools and educators feel responsible for supplying students with food, clothing, dental and medical care, warmth, and safety for their day-to-day survival and to support their potential for growth and ability to learn. They also attempt to provide adequate mental health support to students to address the environmental, community, and household trauma and adversity they could be experiencing. Without prioritizing the importance of providing students with their essential needs, adequate mental health support, and a successful intervention system, the research is clear: students are unable to learn and thrive.

While considering the ACE study and Maslow's hierarchy of needs, understanding the impact of the children's experiences living in communities and crisis areas is critical to understanding the influence it has on students' visible behaviors at school. The role that stress has on children's brain development and cognitive and social growth is often cited as a critical factor in why children living with adverse life experiences perform poorly in school. Stress alters children's language, social, and cognitive development and is not easily controlled by educators because so much of it derives from family life and events outside of school (Jensen, 2009).

Safety concerns, food insecurity, inconsistent living arrangements, and multiple adverse childhood experiences and trauma can make growing, learning, and thriving in school extremely difficult. Many students come to school with abundant stress, mental health challenges, lack of necessities, and multiple ACEs. The situations experienced by students can increase the likelihood of stress, secondary trauma, and compassion fatigue for the teachers and educators who work with them daily. Witnessing such anguish can lead to educator attrition, turnover, and stress.

Related National Trends

The complicated dynamics of teacher stress, secondary trauma, and attrition within the context of schools situated in regions challenged by the opioid crisis are parallel to findings and results of national surveys. Educators leaving the field within a relatively short span due to escalating demands, inadequate support, and unrealistic expectations have been a persistent concern in education (Darling-Hammond et al., 2017; Education Week Research Center, 2023; National Center for Education Statistics, 2023; Ormiston et al., 2022). Recent research highlights the emergence of secondary traumatic stress and compassion fatigue as pivotal factors contributing to teachers' departure (Oberg et al., 2023). Additionally, chronic absenteeism emerges as a pressing concern exacerbated by the intersecting challenges of adverse childhood experiences and the lingering effects of the aftermath of the COVID-19 pandemic. Both teacher attrition and chronic absenteeism are nationwide educational challenges yet are more prominent in schools located in opioid-crisis regions.

Educator Attrition, Stress, and Shortages

Teacher stress and secondary trauma can result in rapid teacher turnover and attrition for schools and districts in opioid-crisis regions. Research suggests that generally, many teachers often leave the field of education within three to five years due to increasing demands, lack of support, and unrealistic expectations from the administration (Darling-Hammond et al., 2017; Education Week Research Center, 2023; National Center for Education Statistics, 2023; Ormiston et al., 2022). Secondary traumatic stress and compassion fatigue are also reasons teachers may leave the profession. As discovered in this investigation, schools located in opioid-crisis regions have educators who are experiencing a concerning level of secondary trauma and stress. Both secondary trauma and compassion fatigue are recognized in the healthcare and mental health fields as reasons why clinicians leave their jobs; it has only recently been addressed in education (Ormiston et al., 2022). As more and more students come to school unprepared to learn due to adverse experiences, trauma, and unmet basic needs, educators' concerns mount, and their well-being and mental health take a toll. Teachers are experiencing added stress and secondary trauma, which impacts their mental health and, unfortunately, leads to medical leave for some. Teacher stress has been linked to significant attrition, contributing to concerns about teacher shortages and the links between turnover and student achievement (Darling-Hammond et al., 2017). The stresses the educators were experiencing in this study, such as student trauma, needs, experiences, parental behaviors, and low Department of Youth Services responses, impact teachers' well-being and teachers in this study voiced concerns about retention. These findings from the research align with the findings and survey results from studies of teachers nationwide.

In 2023, a national teacher survey was commissioned by the Winston School of Education and Social Policy at Merrimack College and conducted by the EdWeek Research Center. The survey results suggest that many teachers feel overworked, underpaid, and under-appreciated, creating potential implications for leaving the teaching profession. Specifically, the survey included 1,178 K-12 teachers across the United States. The results showed that only 20% of teachers are very satisfied with their jobs. Figure 13.1 shows the percentage of teachers who are "very satisfied" with their jobs from 1984 to 2023.

In 2023, just 20% of teachers were very satisfied with their job, compared to 62% in 2008. On a positive note, from 2022 to 2023, teacher satisfaction improved 8%.

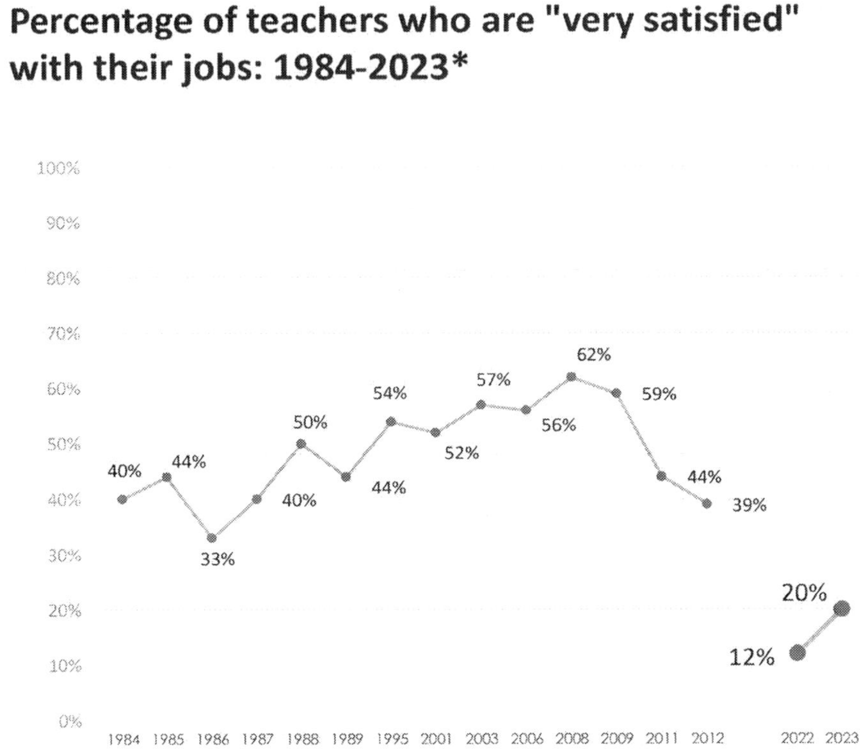

Figure 13.1 Teacher satisfaction

Source: EdWeek Research Center, 2023 Merrimack College Teacher Survey. Reprinted with permissions.

Furthermore, 42% of teachers feel their mental health is having a negative impact on their work. Teachers feel that they are overworked, underpaid, and under-appreciated. In the survey, teachers shared their ideas on how their districts could support their mental well-being. The results are shared in Figure 13.2.

Teachers responded that higher pay, smaller class sizes, discipline support, fewer administrative burdens, acknowledging accomplishments, and encouraging mental health and well-being days were cited as important for mental well-being (Education Week Research Center, 2023).

The research into schools located in opioid-crisis regions suggests that there are challenges to hiring and retaining teachers, especially considering the location of the study was in high-poverty areas with a large number of English language learners and a high percentage of students with disabilities. Literature indicates that staffing challenges disproportionately affect schools in high-poverty areas, English learners, and students with disabilities (Cardichon

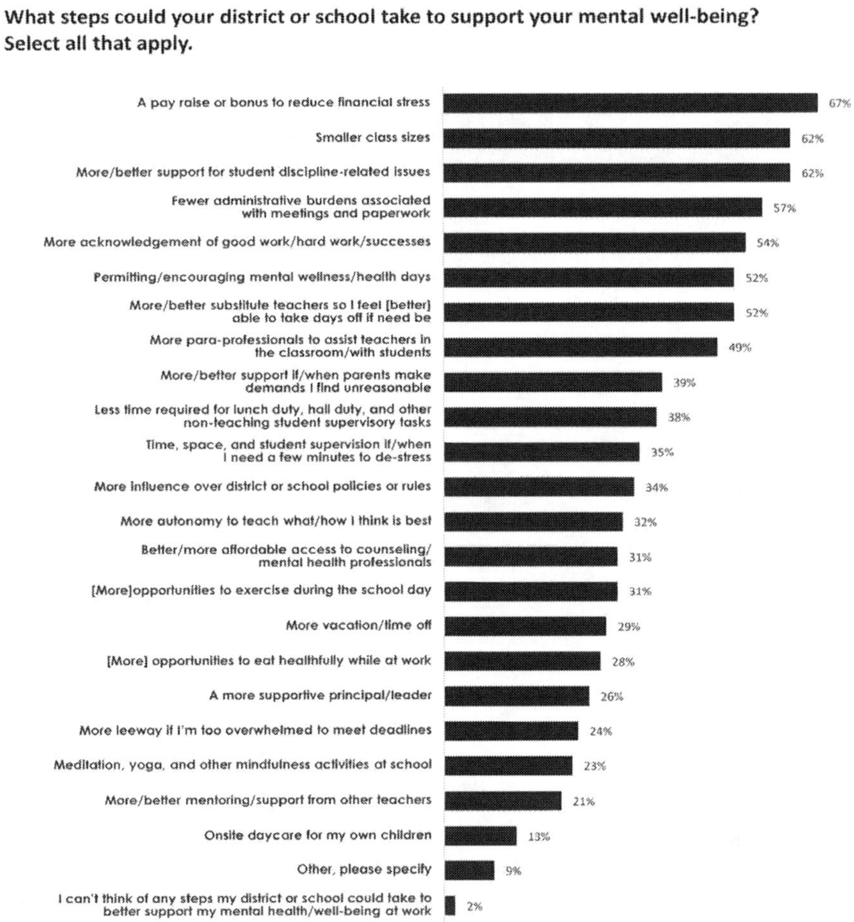

Figure 13.2 How school districts could support teachers' mental well-being

Source: EdWeek Research Center, 2023 Merrimack College Teacher Survey. Reprinted with permissions.

et al., 2020; Goldhaber & Gratz, 2021; Sutcher et al., 2016; U.S. Department of Education, 2023a). High-needs school districts are impacted by teacher attrition to a greater extent than schools with fewer needs and challenges.

The teacher shortage is an issue of national concern, yet it has impacted different types of communities across the country in different ways. A recent survey from the U.S. Department of Education (2023b) reiterated the concerns that schools do not have enough staff to address the issues schools in crisis regions face. Figure 13.3, created by the U.S. Department of Education Raise The Bar Policy Brief (2023a), shows the 2023–2024 projected

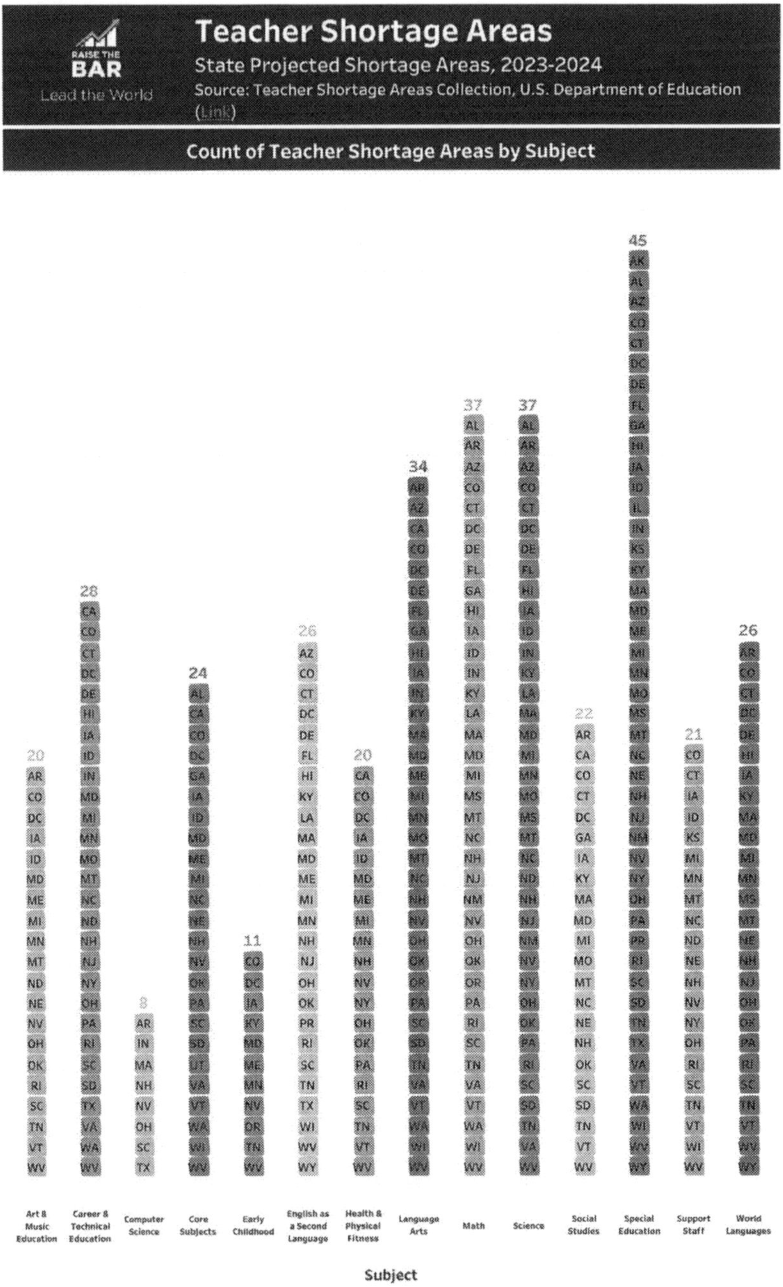

Figure 13.3 Teacher shortage areas

Source: U.S Department of Education (2023): Raise the Bar Policy Brief https://www.ed.gov/raisethebar/Eliminating-Educator-Shortages-through-Increasing-Educator-Diversity

teacher shortages by subject and state. Consequently, for the 2023–2024 school year, leading the country in shortages are special education teachers. Forty-five states anticipated a shortage of qualified special education teachers, and 26 states anticipated a shortage of teachers who are qualified to teach English as a second language (U.S. Department of Education, 2023b). This is a concerning trend given the trajectory of the opioid epidemic and the possibility of increased special education needs in opioid crisis areas. There will be a continued need for special education and disability specialist until the epidemic takes a positive turn.

Unfortunately, this shortage is not specific to just teachers but to other staff as well. As of August 2023, 86% of schools nationwide reported struggling to hire teachers, and 83% said they were struggling to fill other positions like classroom teaching assistants, transportation staff, and mental health professionals (National Center for Education Statistics, 2023). States nationwide were also experiencing shortages of support professionals, such as school language pathologists, occupational therapists, physical therapists, psychologists, nurses, and social workers (Prothero & Riser-Kositsky, 2022). All of the suggested staffing challenges are positions that are needed in opioid-crisis regions to help support students thrive.

In addition to teacher shortages and attrition, chronic absenteeism is another challenging situation for schools in opioid-crisis regions amplified by the COVID-19 pandemic. Unfortunately, this is a national crisis.

Chronic Absenteeism Across the United States

ACEs are linked with high chronic absenteeism rates in school-age children (Stempel et al., 2017). Students who miss 10% of the school year or 18 days for any reason, including excused and unexcused absences, are considered chronically absent. In addition to ACEs, reasons and causes of chronic absenteeism include both out-of-school factors and in-school factors. Out-of-school factors are related to economic disadvantage and health, while in school factors include school climate, safety, instruction, discipline, and student support (Dee, 2023; Gottfried & Hutt, 2019; Rafa, 2017). Nauer (2014) and her team from A Better Picture of Poverty explored the connection between social support and chronic absenteeism. Findings show that students who miss school are significantly impacted by poverty and dysfunctional schools.

Patterns of chronic absenteeism reflect equity issues that are present in opioid-crisis regions and school districts. For example, students who come from low-income families, students with disabilities, and students in the juvenile justice system are more likely to be chronically absent than those who are not. Other reasons include unsafe schools, bullying, homelessness, housing instability, and substance use, which can impact students' attendance (Nostrand-Nauer et al., 2014). Schools located in opioid-crisis regions

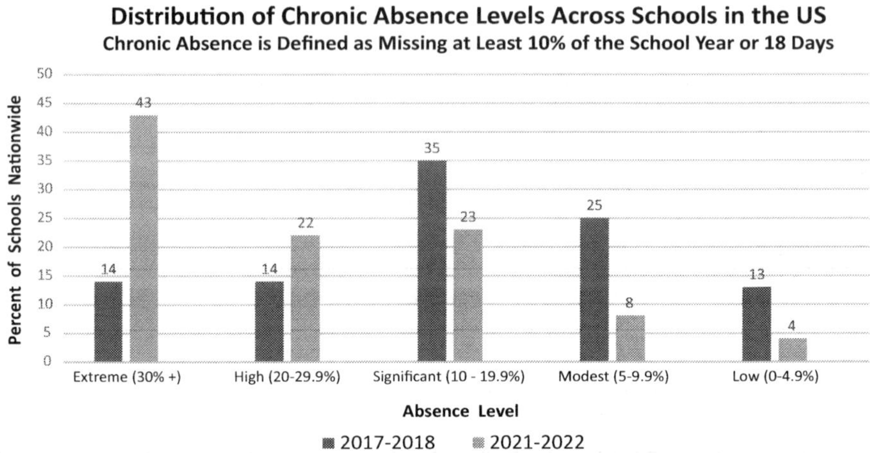

Figure 13.4 Distribution of chronic absence levels across schools

Source: Rising Tide of Chronic Absence Challenges Schools, Attendance Works and the Everyone Graduates Center at Johns Hopkins University, October, 2023. Recreated with Permission

have been challenged by ACEs and both school and out-of-school factors that have led to chronic absenteeism.

Unfortunately, this is not only a challenge in opioid-crisis regions, but since COVID-19, this is also a challenge across the United States. The distribution of chronic absence levels across the United States is illustrated in Figure 13.4.

According to an analysis from Attendance Works and Everyone Graduates Center at Johns Hopkins University (2023), there is a fivefold increase in the percentage of elementary and middle school students who have extreme rates of absence, and 30% of students are chronically absent. These national trends align with the findings of the research and most likely are exacerbated in opioid-crisis regions due to the already present challenges.

Big Picture and Interventions

The impact the opioid epidemic has on schools located in crisis regions is an adaptive challenge without one clear solution. However, awareness of the complexity and challenges associated with this public health emergency is necessary to start understanding the effect of the crisis and how it influences educators, schools, and students. Comprehending the issues through the lens of the schools and the perspectives of educators is powerful in understanding the prevailing impact.

According to the results of this research, there is no consistency and no coherent plan in place. According to participants' perceptions, states, districts, and schools seem to have the autonomy to make their own decisions and launch individualized plans and initiatives to combat this public health crisis within their schools. Since there is no federally guided plan, school districts seem reactive versus proactive in addressing this ongoing challenge. Furthermore, the impact the COVID-19 pandemic has had on schools has expanded and added to the already preexisting concerns in opioid-crisis regions, such as students attending school with unmet basic needs, student trauma and mental health challenges, teacher shortages, and chronic absenteeism.

Combining the Research

Before exploring the proposed solutions, it is essential to first present an overarching summary or "big picture" of the discoveries, contextualizing them with respect to each component. Employing the educational institution as a focal point for comprehending the opioid epidemic, Figure 13.5 merges literature, the theoretical framework (adverse childhood experience study), research findings, and insights from educators. This visualization serves to emphasize the impact on students and educators facing a crisis.

The impact demonstrated unpacks the challenges educators are enduring, such as students' unmet basic needs and adverse childhood experiences leading to a diagnosed disability, traumas, and other direct impacts on schools. The consequential impact result is a sharp shift in the school's responsibilities. Schools are attempting solutions to meet the needs of the diverse population; however, the needs outweigh the solutions. A snapshot of solutions,

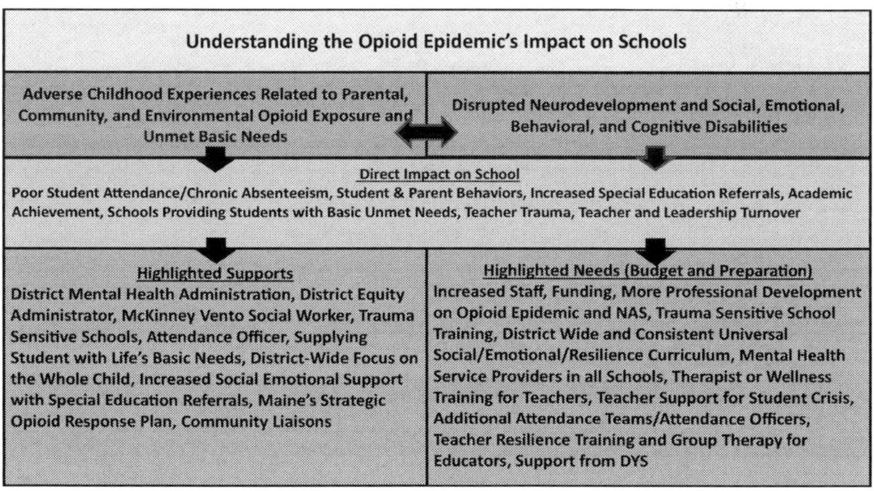

Figure 13.5 Understanding the opioid epidemic's impact on schools

highlighted supports, and additional needs discussed in Chapter 10 are also illustrated in Figure 13.5, combining the broad findings.

At the core, many students are attending school with unmet basic needs and complications of adverse childhood experiences, resulting in an abundance of consequential impacts on the school and educators working in the schools.

The results delineated are connected, and there is an evident snowball effect between students, teachers, schools, district leadership, and society throughout this study. Table 13.6 establishes the relationship between the opioid epidemic as a societal health crisis and the impact on the district leadership, school, teachers, and students.

Table 13.6 Relationship between opioid epidemic and impact on education

Student
Opioid Epidemic and Impact on the Student Adverse home and community factors are associated with lost learning opportunities. Students come to school with an abundance of stress, mental health challenges, lack of necessities, and adverse childhood experiences that impact learning and those in contact with them in school.
School
Opioid Epidemic Impact on School and Learning A significant number of students in opioid-crisis regions are living in poverty and are experiencing homelessness, transiency, neglect, and caregiver instability. Additionally, grandparents and other family members, guardians, or family friends are raising children, children are experiencing trauma, and basic needs are unmet. Those outside factors impact attendance, tardiness, behaviors, academic achievement at school, educator resilience, and mental health. Additionally, teacher retention is a possible concern.
Schools Are Responsible for Providing Students With Basic Needs Educators report that many students in opioid-crisis regions could possibly be experiencing neglect because of parental drug abuse, home instability, and poverty. Schools are responsible for providing students with basic unmet needs, such as food, water, clothing, warmth, sleep, dental, medical, and safety. Children are unable to learn if their basic needs are unmet. Therefore, to learn and thrive, schools have taken on that additional responsibility.
Teacher
Opioid Epidemic and Impact on the Teacher Teachers are experiencing added stress and secondary trauma, impacting their mental health and leading to medical leaves for some. Others are leaving the district they are working in and the teaching profession entirely. The impact on student learning, adverse childhood experiences, and providing students with unmet basic needs impacts teachers' mental health. Student trauma, needs, experiences, parental behaviors, and challenges with Department of Youth Services responses have been cited as negatively impacting teachers' well-being.

District Leadership

Proactive Preparation

Lack of organizational systems and proactive preparation result in inadequate support for schools, teachers, and students. Inadequate support can lead to failing schools, teacher attrition, and turnover.

Consistency

Different schools within districts have inconsistent solutions, curriculums, and initiatives.

Implementing social-emotional, trauma-informed, and resilience curricula is inconsistent from school to school within districts. Lack of consistency is problematic when students are transient, frequently attending various schools in the same district.

Funding

There is a vast disconnect between what administrators, educators, and students need and the funding available to obtain those needs.

Society

Adverse Childhood Experiences Related to Opioid Epidemic

Children's exposure to the opioid epidemic and related environmental stressors increases the likelihood of adverse childhood experiences and unmet basic needs. Federal funding, policymakers, and community support are necessary to address these issues at the core.

This cycle will continue unless solutions are made available and policies change to add additional support in schools and the surrounding community. The cycle is an adaptive challenge that has been uncovered but not adequately addressed.

Table 13.6 illustrates a complex interplay of factors stemming from the opioid epidemic. Adverse home and community factors linked to the opioid epidemic result in challenges for students, including stress, mental health issues, and unmet basic needs. Students bring these challenges into the school environment, affecting attendance, behavior, academic achievement, and teacher resilience. Schools take on the added responsibility of addressing students' unmet basic needs due to external factors such as neglect resulting from parental drug abuse. This results in teacher strain. The impact of the opioid epidemic on students, coupled with the responsibility of addressing unmet basic needs, contributes to increased stress and secondary trauma for teachers.

Teacher retention is affected, with some leaving the district or the profession. Student challenges and teacher impact result in district leadership challenges. Lack of organizational systems and proactive preparation at the district level leads to inadequate support for schools, teachers, and students. Inconsistencies in solutions and curriculums across schools within districts pose challenges, especially for transient students, and funding disparities further exacerbate the difficulties administrators, educators, and students face.

Teacher, students, and school district challenges have societal implications because the opioid epidemic contributes to adverse childhood experiences and unmet basic needs among children, and from there, the cycle repeats because of the relationship each aspect has with each other. Society's response, including federal funding, policymaker involvement, and community support, is essential to address these core issues.

The themes are interconnected because the challenges faced by students have a cascading effect on schools and teachers. Inadequate support at the district level exacerbates issues within schools and classrooms. Inconsistencies across schools hinder effective responses to student needs, highlighting the importance of a unified approach. Finally, societal factors, including policies and community support, play a pivotal role in breaking the cycle of challenges related to the opioid epidemic.

In summary, the relationship between these points emphasizes the need for a comprehensive and coordinated approach involving students, schools, teachers, district leadership, and broader societal efforts to address the multifaceted challenges arising from the opioid epidemic.

Further investigation should focus on solutions and interventions.

Bringing It All Together

This chapter explores the complex challenges faced by schools, educators, and students in areas affected by the opioid epidemic. It emphasizes the interconnected nature of these challenges, ranging from unmet basic needs for students to the secondary trauma experienced by teachers. Adverse home and community factors linked to the opioid epidemic contribute to lost learning opportunities, placing the onus on schools to address basic needs and increasing stress for educators. The connection of the finding to current national trends is clear particularly in relationship to teacher shortages, teacher stress, and chronic absenteeism. Teacher retention is a critical concern due to the strain caused by students' challenges, adverse experiences, and unmet needs. District leadership faces challenges such as inadequate support structures and inconsistent solutions. The societal implications accentuate the need for federal funding, policymaker involvement, and community support.

References

Attendance Works. (2023). *Rising tide of chronic absence challenges schools.* https://www.attendanceworks.org/rising-tide-of-chronic-absence-challenges-schools/

and supplemental spreadsheet: https://docs.google.com/spreadsheets/d/15yNTUUNwHzhFjQRCYgY5o7KE5pGoVFtk/edit#gid=1137911798

Berliner, D. (2009). Are teachers responsible for low achievement by poor students? *Kappa Delta Pi*, *75*, 4–8.

Cardichon, J., Darling-Hammond, L., Yang, M., Scott, C., Shields, P. M., & Burns, D. (2020, February 12). *Inequitable opportunity to learn: Student access to certified and experienced teachers*. Learning Policy Institute. https://learningpolicyinstitute.org/product/crdc-teacher-access-report.

Centers for Disease Control and Prevention. (2014). *The ACE pyramid*. National Center for Injury Prevention and Control, Division of Violence Prevention. https://www.cdc.gov/violenceprevention/acestudy/about.html

Darling-Hammond, L., Sutcher, L., & Carver Thomas, D. (2017, November 17). *Why addressing teacher turnover matters* [Blog]. Learning Policy Institute. https://learningpolicyinstitute.org/blog/why-addressing-teacher-turnover-matters

Dee, T. (2023). *Higher chronic absenteeism threatens academic recovery from the COVID-19 pandemic*. Center for Open Science. https://osf.io/bfg3p/

Drescher, J., Steyer, L., Townley-Flores, C., & Humphreys, K. (2022). Has the opioid crisis affected student learning? A national analysis of growth rates. *The ANNALS of the American Academy of Political and Social Science*, *703*(1), 234–261. https://doi.org/10.1177/00027162231151524

Goldhaber, D., & Gratz, T. (2021). *School district staffing challenges in a rapidly recovering economy*. Center for Analysis of Longitudinal Data in Education Research. https://caldercenter.org/publications/school-district-staffing-challenges-rapidly-recovering-economy.

Gottfried, M. A., & Hutt, E. L. (2019). *Absent from school: Understanding and addressing student absenteeism*. Harvard Education Press.

Jensen, E. (2009). *Teaching with poverty in mind: What being poor does to kids' brains and what schools can do about it*. Association for Supervision and Curriculum Development.

Maslow, A. H. (1968). *Toward a psychology of being*. (2nd ed.). Van.

Education Week Research Center. (2023). *Merrimack College Winston School of Education and Social Policy*. National teacher survey. https://www.merrimack.edu/academics/education-and-social-policy/about/merrimack-college-teacher-survey/[0]

National Center for Educational Statistics. (2023). *U.S. Department of Education*. https://nces.ed.gov/

Nauer, K., Mader, N., Robinson, G., & Jacobs, T., with Cory, B., Moss J., and Bloodworth A. (2014). A Better Picture of Poverty What Chronic Absenteeism and Risk Load Reveal About NYC's Lowest-Income Elementary Schools. Retrieved From: https://www.attendanceworks.org/wp-content/uploads/2017/06/BetterPictureofPoverty_PA_FINAL_001.pdf

Nostrand-Nauer, K., Mader, N., Robinson, G., & Jacobs, T. (2014). *A better picture of poverty: What chronic absenteeism and risk load reveal about NYC's lowest-income elementary schools*. The New School Center for New York City Affairs. www.attendanceworks.org/wordpress/wp-content/uploads/2014/11/BetterPictureofPoverty_PA_FINAL_001.pdf.

Oberg, G., Carroll, A., & Macmahon, S. (2023). Compassion fatigue and secondary traumatic stress in teachers: How they contribute to burnout and how they are related to trauma-awareness. *Frontiers in Education*, *8*, 1128618. https://doi.org/10.3389/feduc.2023.1128618

Ormiston, H. E., Nygaard, M. A., & Apgar, S. (2022). A systematic review of secondary traumatic stress and compassion fatigue in teachers. *School Mental Health, 14*, 802–817.

Prothero, A., & Riser-Kositsky, M. (2022). *School counselors and psychologists remain scarce even as needs rise*. Education Week. https://www.edweek.org/leadership/school-counselors-and-psychologists-remain-scarce-even-as-needs-rise/2022/03.

Rafa, A. (2017). *Chronic absenteeism: A key indicator of student success. Policy analysis*. Education Commission of the States.

Stempel, H., Cox-Martin, M., Bronsert, M., Dickinson, L. M., & Allison, M. A. (2017). Chronic school absenteeism and the role of adverse childhood experiences. *Academic Pediatrics, 17*(8), 837–843. https://doi.org/10.1016/j.acap.2017.09.013

Sutcher, L., Darling-Hammond, L., & Carver-Thomas, D. (2016*). A coming crisis in teaching? Teacher supply, demand, and shortages in the U.S.* Learning Policy Institute. https://learningpolicyinstitute.org/product/coming-crisis-teaching.

U.S. Department of Education. (2023a). *Raising the bar policy brief.* https://www.ed.gov/raisethebar/Eliminating-Educator-Shortages-through-Increasing-Educator-Diversity#_ftn38

U.S. Department of Education. (2023b). *Teacher shortage area data, 2023–24.* https://tsa.ed.gov/#/home/

14 Conclusion and Further Exploration

Collaborative Interventions for Resilience and Systematic Change Designed for Schools in Opioid-Crisis Regions

> Districts and schools are woefully unprepared. We are woefully unprepared. When I supervised child find before I was the principal here, in one year three years ago, we brought in more than 400 preschoolers for evaluation. Most of those young children were evaluated because there was a substance abuse issue when mom was pregnant. We knew that three years ago. Three years ago! We have not prepared for those children in our district. We know, but we are not addressing the needs of those children in our schools, and we are still not preparing for them. . . . We have not prepared ourselves for the surge of students impacted by the opioid epidemic. Our response is terrible, but I do not think you will find a place prepared for this. How can you prepare for this? We are all just running on a shoestring.
>
> – Pat, New Hampshire Principal

Within opioid-crisis regions, schools have a powerful opportunity for transformation.

Beyond the challenges, there lie incredible stories of resilience and unwavering dedication. Educators go above and beyond traditional roles to nurture their students' fundamental needs and safety.

Their stories reveal a profound understanding of the daily realities students face where trauma and instability often, and understandably, overshadow learning. Yet, within these difficulties, educators are rising as frontline responders, providing education and essential support, from clothing to food to emotional care, and creating safe havens within their classrooms, filling the gaps left by systemic shortcomings.

Despite their overwhelming burdens, teachers continue to represent resilience and selflessness. Their commitment to ensuring not just academic growth but also the well-being and safety of their students is evidence of their profound empathy and dedication. Their tireless efforts, fueled by care for their students, shine amidst adversity, exemplifying educators' incredible impact beyond textbooks and lesson plans. Their unwavering belief in the potential of their students, coupled with their endless acts of kindness,

DOI: 10.4324/9781003378204-17

illuminates a path of hope and resilience within communities facing the harsh realities of the opioid crisis.

Their commitment is inspiring, but it's also crucial to acknowledge the toll this crisis takes on their well-being. Their dedication to their students is admirable, but the toll on their own mental health is undeniable. The unexpected development of secondary trauma among educators demands further attention and support. Their stories and experiences call for a deeper understanding of the impact on educators' mental health and well-being while advocating for systemic support to lessen their burdens.

Although the impact on teachers needs to be illuminated, this isn't a story of despair; it's a call for collective action and systemic change. The findings of this research point to the next steps, further investigations, and, most importantly, reveal possible interventions and solutions to address some of these profound systematic gaps.

Communities, policymakers, and educators should unite to create inspiring and hopeful next steps where schools become resilient communities, addressing students' academic needs and mental health challenges. By implementing trauma-informed practices, fostering holistic collaborations, providing extended wraparound services, partnering with community agencies, and providing comprehensive mental health support for both students and educators, together, we can begin to pave the way for a brighter future.

Interventions

The educational landscape constantly evolves, and addressing the multifaceted challenges students face inside and outside the classroom is imperative. We have an exciting opportunity to tackle the diverse challenges. It's crucial to dive into key aspects of enhancing professional growth, bolstering support networks, and implementing broader systemic changes within school districts to cultivate an even more nurturing and effective learning atmosphere for our students.

Various interventions emerged from this exploratory research and follow-up studies, reflecting the essential needs identified by participants. Nationwide, some school districts have started implementing several of these strategies, while others have minimal support, and many do not know where to start. Some suggestions require a robust and time-consuming overhaul that may not be feasible for some districts, while other interventions can be implemented immediately.

These interventions offer promising pathways for further exploration. Consider these 18 proposed supports, innovative solutions, and interventions as potential further investigations that can be embraced, refined, and evaluated to measure effective integration and impact on our educational landscape.

Interventions in Schools – Educators and District Leadership

1. **Targeted Professional Development:** Neonatal Abstinence Syndrome (NAS) and exposure to adverse childhood experiences (ACEs) can require mental health care, are associated with disabilities, and may require additional school interventions. Educators need targeted professional development in NAS and ACEs to comprehend students' challenges and cognitive and behavioral disabilities and identify necessary accommodations within the classroom setting. This should be a focus of not only special education teachers but also all teachers in the district. One of the findings is that it could take months for students to receive recommended special education services due to attendance inconsistencies and chasing parents for approval signatures; therefore, in the meantime, all teachers are responsible and need the tools for success. This requires not only awareness but also a proactive approach to ensure students receive the support they need to thrive academically despite the challenges posed by opioid exposure.
2. **Create Trauma-Sensitive Learning Environments:** Educators can effectively support students by guiding them to recognize how their experiences shape their behavior, thoughts, and emotions. Equipping teachers with tools and resources enables them to assist students in establishing a sense of security, safety, and optimism. Encouraging reflective thinking during times of intense emotions aids in the healing process for students enduring traumatic situations. Additionally, fostering a trauma-sensitive learning environment teaches educators the significance of remaining composed when dealing with students experiencing emotional distress. Trauma-sensitive training is designed to educate educators, offering insights and strategies rooted in trauma awareness to navigate these situations with sensitivity and understanding.
3. **Administrative Training on Social-Emotional Learning and Trauma-Informed Practices:** Findings suggest that in some school districts, teachers are more frequently provided with training on social-emotional learning and trauma-informed practices, but the school principals and district administration do not have training in these areas. Administration plays a pivotal role in shaping the overall school culture and policies. Having administrators trained in SEL and trauma-informed practices ensures a more cohesive and consistent approach to student support.
4. **School-Wide Protocols:** When students share adversity, trauma, and other situations, educators report a feeling of helplessness, not knowing what to do, while often feeling that their requests and pleas for help go unanswered. Give educators the tools to know where to go for help, specifically providing detailed steps and expectations with names,

numbers, and guidance. By creating a school or district protocol for serious student reports needing crisis interventions, educators have a plan to move forward, hopefully alleviating some of their anxiety, stress, and feelings of helplessness. In addition, providing educators with foundational knowledge on addressing mental health needs will be helpful when students share such situations. This holistic approach acknowledges the interconnectedness of mental health and academic success, fostering a more compassionate and effective learning environment for both the students and the educators.

5. **Mental Health and First Aid Training:** In conjunction with schoolwide protocols shared above, provide educators with opportunities to acquire a mental health and first aid certification. Typically, the certification includes a training course that teaches health and substance-use issues.
6. **Guided Group Therapy and Resilience Workshops for Educators:** Investing in the well-being of teachers and school staff is essential to creating a resilient educational community. Providing resilience training, professionally guided group therapy, conflict resolution workshops, and wellness trainers can contribute to a healthier, more supportive school culture. This investment not only benefits individual educators but also positively impacts the overall educational experience for students. Teachers are experiencing some significant trauma and may not be aware that other educators in the same schools are experiencing the same feelings, emotions, and heartaches. Knowing that they have each other as a support system and giving them the tools to address their own mental health could create a supportive community and potentially address issues of teacher attrition and improve retention.
7. **Consistent District-Wide Resilience and Social-Emotional Programs and Curriculum:** Participants stressed the significance of implementing a district-wide resilience and social-emotional curriculum. The idea is to have a unified program across the district, ensuring consistency in language, strategies, and expectations as students transition between schools and progress through various grade levels. The rationale is that when schools have autonomy in choosing or creating their own curriculum, there is a notable lack of consistency. This approach requires students to adapt to new program language, tools, and expectations each academic year or with every inter-district school move. And as the research shows, students move frequently between schools. A unified program would alleviate student stress.
8. **Parental Relationship Building and Conflict Resolution Workshops:** The research revealed that relationship building with parents is difficult. The results also suggest that it is difficult to de-escalate parents and situations that arise. Training and workshops on relationship building with

parents, conflict resolution, and de-escalating skills would prepare teachers and administrators with some "tools" to address such challenges.

9. **Clinical Interdisciplinary Intervention Teams:** Participants also emphasized the importance of mental health workers, community resources, nurses, and social workers. Creating clinical interdisciplinary intervention teams, including mental health providers, community members, nurses, teachers, and social workers designed to collaborate and support students and families in need. These teams would meet in school, create individual plans for students in need, and would be an added layer of support in addition to the academic teams working within the schools. These clinical teams would focus on students' social, emotional, and behavioral needs and transitions from school to home.
10. **Mental Health Administrator:** To oversee and support the district's school-based social workers, mental health providers, and interdisciplinary clinical intervention teams. The administrator's role contributes to implementing trauma-informed practices and SEL initiatives across all schools within the district. The director guides interventions addressing social/emotional and behavioral needs, fostering collaboration with the school's social workers, social-emotional learning coach, and administrative personnel.
11. **Prepare Future Teachers for the Reality of Today's Classrooms:** Recognizing the pressing need for more teachers and the reality of teacher attrition, especially in the face of a national teacher shortage crisis, there should be an emphasis on adequately preparing college students enrolled in teacher preparation programs. This preparation would equip them to navigate potential exposure to trauma and empower them with effective action steps when faced with challenging situations. The goal is to mitigate potential attrition linked to unpreparedness and foster a more resilient teaching workforce. Train future teachers in the tools that are needed to address student ACEs, trauma, and associated disabilities. Also, provide future teachers with resilience training, conflict resolution workshops, and relationship-building classes. The findings of this study reveal that multiple teachers ($N = 7$) with five or less years of experience voiced concern that they were not taught about trauma and adversity and how to navigate such situations in their teacher preparation programs.

Interventions in Schools – Students

12. **Student Support Groups:** Student-led or adult-led (depending on the age and grade of students) support groups for students who have family members struggling with opioid addiction offer valuable benefits by

providing a peer support network that reduces isolation and combats the stigma associated with addiction. The supportive community helps alleviate guilt and shame while educating students about addiction. The networking opportunities within these groups should also connect participants with mental health providers and offer community resources. These at-school support groups would contribute to a holistic approach to address some of their emotional and practical needs while reducing isolation and stigmas associated with addiction.

13. **Toolbox Project:** In Chapter 10, the Toolbox Project was introduced (refer to Visual 10.6). As referred by 83% of the interview participants who worked in New Hampshire, it is worth mentioning as a suggested intervention tool. The goal of the ToolBox Project was to provide tools to reinforce resilience for students who may need them and provide a visual reference throughout the day. Interview participants credited the Toolbox Project Program as a successful calming process to avoid a crisis while minimizing explosive behaviors in the school. The poster (shown in Figure 14.1) lists tools for learning and tools for life. The poster should be displayed in every classroom, hallway, office, and cafeteria. When students are overwhelmed, challenged, angry, sad, or frustrated, staff points to the posted "Toolbox" so that students can decide how to react to their feelings using the suggested "tools." Depending on the situation, the student will use an appropriate tool to address the issue or feeling they are experiencing (The Toolbox Project, n.d.).

Interventions – Policy, Community, and Leadership

14. **Department of Youth Services Integrated Approach:** Creating a strong system or protocol that fosters effective communication between schools and the Department of Youth Services is essential. Exploring the option of employing DYS workers or forming a dedicated DYS Team for each district or school could be a solution to resolve the communication and response gap between schools and such departments. This proactive measure aims to expedite responses, especially when a child is perceived as in crisis, and the child returning home may not be the most advisable course of action.
15. **Community Resources Available in School:** The research revealed that many families are unaware of the community support and resources available, and some families reject resources because they do not want community employees or others coming to their homes. Schools should collaborate with community programs and resources frequently, ensuring that these resources are seamlessly integrated into the school environment. Having those resources available in schools and creating

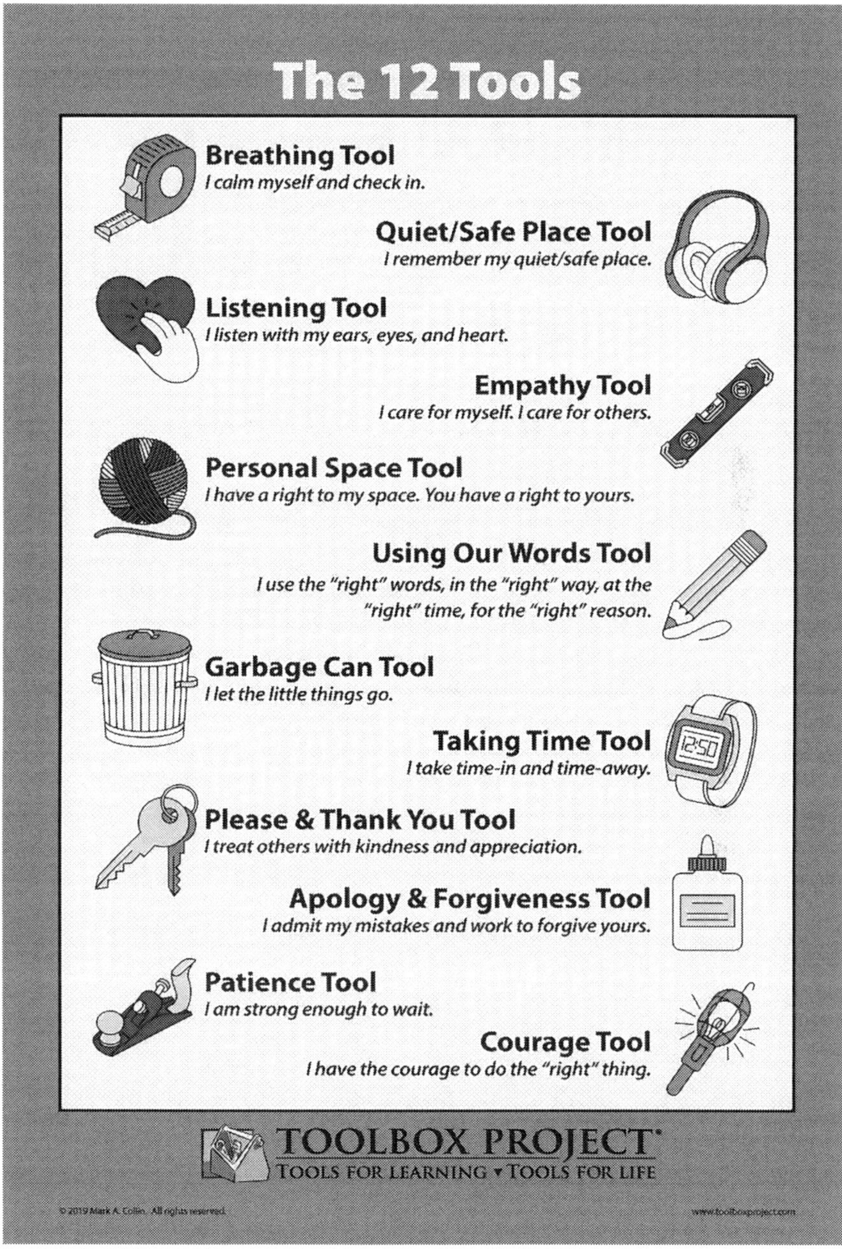
The 12 Tools
Breathing Tool
I calm myself and check in.
Quiet/Safe Place Tool
I remember my quiet/safe place.
Listening Tool
I listen with my ears, eyes, and heart.
Empathy Tool
I care for myself. I care for others.
Personal Space Tool
I have a right to my space. You have a right to yours.
Using Our Words Tool
I use the "right" words, in the "right" way, at the "right" time, for the "right" reason.
Garbage Can Tool
I let the little things go.
Taking Time Tool
I take time-in and time-away.
12:50
Please & Thank You Tool
I treat others with kindness and appreciation.
Apology & Forgiveness Tool
I admit my mistakes and work to forgive yours.
Patience Tool
I am strong enough to wait.
Courage Tool
I have the courage to do the "right" thing.
TOOLBOX PROJECT
TOOLS FOR LEARNING • TOOLS FOR LIFE
© 2019 Mark A. Collin. All rights reserved.
www.toolboxproject.com

Figure 14.1 The toolbox

community partnerships will give the children in the schools more access to the available community tools and resources.

16. **Standardization for Student Tracking:** Establishing uniform policies for students transitioning between schools within the same district, across districts, within states, and across state borders is crucial. This uniformity is vital to guarantee a smooth educational progression for students, minimizing the impact of administrative variations and tracking system disparities. Furthermore, it is imperative to proactively address the distinctive challenges homeless students face, such as improving transportation options and tracking systems to enhance their educational access without the potential of getting lost in the system.

The findings suggest that, although the government monitors and establishes norms for educating homeless children, districts lack consistency in implementing McKinney-Vento initiatives and tracking homeless populations. Some districts have a person designated for this role in each of their neighborhood schools, supported by an attendance team and truancy officers. Other districts have one person per district monitoring homeless populations in school systems with 10,000-plus students. Other districts assign an already-overwhelmed staff member to take on this role or even worse some districts just add the words McKinney-Vento to a person's job description for compliance. Achieving uniformity in these efforts across districts and states can help mitigate the challenges faced by students who may otherwise encounter difficulties, get lost within the system, or find themselves in dangerous situations while relocating throughout the United States. Developing a standardized homeless protocol and tracking system, along with consistent positions and policies across states, can ensure that students experiencing homelessness are appropriately monitored and provided for.

17. **Residential Public School Model:** Participants emphasized the significance of before-school programs and after-school programs and providing breakfast, lunch, and dinner in schools, stating that the longer students stay in school, the safer they are. In light of difficulties with the Department of Youth Services, establishing residential public schools in crisis-prone areas would guarantee students' safety, well-being, nourishment, and support. Collaboration with community services and leveraging existing resources could pave the way for a novel educational model, consolidating all essential elements in one location to establish a secure haven for students to develop, flourish, and learn.
18. **Multi-Sectoral Approach:** Create a multi-sectoral approach to mitigate the adverse impacts of opioid-use disorders on health, public welfare, and the economy. Using Maine Opioid Response (2023) as a guide, focus on infrastructure, prevention, public safety, harm reduction,

treatment, and recovery. Specifically, in the prevention domain, the plan targets schools with six strategies: ensuring access to Pre-K for all children, promoting awareness of childhood brain development and substance-use disorders, expanding behavioral health support in schools, advocating for policies to prevent early substance use, fostering local partnerships for primary prevention initiatives, and investing in secondary prevention efforts to identify and support high-risk youth. These strategies encompass a range of measures, from early childhood development support to community engagement and education, all aimed at reducing the incidence of substance-use disorders.

Further Investigations

The research, overall, served as an exploration study that provided valuable insights, paving the way for continued investigation and inquiry. Numerous themes emerged during this project, each representing a unique phenomenon deserving deeper exploration. The possibilities for in-depth understanding are abundant, from attendance and teacher trauma to student behaviors, parent involvement and behaviors, and the impacts on special education. The dynamics of transiency, family interactions, student resilience, community involvement, and the effects of leadership and teacher turnover all contribute to ideas for potential research, and these are just a few.

Moreover, the scope of further investigations may extend to comprehend crucial aspects such as longitudinal studies of different geographical locations of schools in crisis regions, a national collection of district solutions to compile and explore, and the rural impacts of the opioid epidemic on schools. As we continue to navigate this public health emergency, the need for further investigation becomes increasingly evident, especially in the face of the ongoing opioid epidemic and its impacts on children, schools and educators. This urgency emphasizes the need for knowledge and understanding to effectively address the far-reaching consequences of this adaptive challenge, ultimately paving the way for a hopeful future.

Bringing It All Together

The insights gained from this research offer valuable solutions to overcome the challenges posed by the opioid crisis. Of course, many of the suggestions require funding, manpower and support. The educational realm, affected by this crisis, benefits greatly from a united and comprehensive strategy. Prioritizing professional growth, mental health support, and collective initiatives within districts presents an opportunity to cultivate an environment that promotes academic success and well-being for students and educators. Recognizing the interconnectedness of individuals, systems, and schools, a collaborative effort involving policymakers, educators, and communities emerges as the key to tackling the multi-dimensional issues presented by the opioid crisis. Together, through these concerted efforts, schools can transform into resilient communities equipped to navigate the complexities of not only the opioid crisis but also other challenges impacting students today.

In conclusion, schools in opioid-crisis regions find themselves at the crossroads of challenge and opportunity. The stories of resilience and dedication among educators unfold as they address students' fundamental needs and safety, creating safe havens within their classrooms. Despite overwhelming burdens, teachers exemplify unwavering commitment, empathy, and selflessness in adversity. However, it is essential to recognize the toll on their well-being and advocate for systemic support to support teachers and provide students with the opportunities to learn and thrive. Comprehensive interventions for further exploration are offered in this chapter, ranging from targeted professional development to a multi-sectoral approach, aiming to transform schools into resilient communities that address academic and mental health needs. The collective interventions highlight the importance of collaboration among communities, policymakers, and educators to foster a nurturing and effective learning atmosphere for students facing the harsh realities of the opioid crisis and beyond.

References

Maine Opioid Response: 2023–2025 Strategic Action Plan. (2023). *Maine Governor's office of policy innovation and the future.* https://www.maine.gov/future/sites/maine.gov.future/files/2023-08/GOPIF_OpioidReport_2023_exsum_digital_0.pdf

The ToolBox Project. (n.d.). *Tools for learning. Tools for life.* https://toolboxproject.com/

Index

Note: Page numbers in *italics* indicate a figure and page numbers in **bold** indicate a table on the corresponding page.

Made in the USA
Las Vegas, NV
19 September 2026

a8cd18f1-74a8-4604-b8ac-8f8182e8e896R01